JOURNAL OF MEDICAL S

VOICES

Collected Essays on Language, Laughter, and Life

LEONARD L. LAPOINTE, PHD

EDITOR-IN-CHIEF
Journal of Medical Speech-Language Pathology

FACULTY
Francis Eppes Distinguished Professor of Communication Science & Disorders
College of Communication and Information

Associate Faculty: Program in Neuroscience
Associate Faculty: College of Medicine
Florida State University

CO-DIRECTOR
TMH-FSU Neurolinguistic-Neurocognitive Research Center
Tallahassee Memorial Hospital

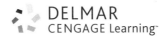

Australia • Brazil • Japan • Korea • Mexico • Singapore • Spain • United Kingdom • United States

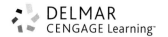
DELMAR
CENGAGE Learning

Journal of Medical Speech-Language Pathology:
Voices: Collected Essays on Language, Laughter, and Life
Leonard L. LaPointe, PhD

Vice President, Career and Professional Editorial:
Dave Garza

Director of Learning Solutions:
Matthew Kane

Senior Acquisitions Editor:
Sherry Dickinson

Managing Editor:
Marah Bellegarde

Product Manager:
Natalie Pashoukos

Editorial Assistant:
Anthony Souza

Vice President, Career and Professional Marketing:
Jennifer McAvey

Marketing Director:
Wendy Mapstone

Marketing Manager:
Kristin McNary

Marketing Coordinator:
Scott Chrysler

Production Director:
Carolyn Miller

Production Manager:
Andrew Crouth

Senior Content Project Manager:
James Zayicek

Project Manager:
Pre-PressPMG

Senior Art Director:
David Arsenault

© 2010 Delmar, Cengage Learning

ALL RIGHTS RESERVED. No part of this work covered by the copyright herein may be reproduced, transmitted, stored or used in any form or by any means graphic, electronic, or mechanical, including but not limited to photocopying, recording, scanning, digitizing, taping, Web distribution, information networks, or information storage and retrieval systems, except as permitted under Section 107 or 108 of the 1976 United States Copyright Act, without the prior written permission of the publisher.

For product information and technology assistance,
contact us at **Cengage Learning
Customer & Sales Support, 1-800-354-9706**

For permission to use material from this text or product,
submit all requests online at **cengage.com/permissions**
Further permissions questions can be emailed to
permissionrequest@cengage.com

Library of Congress Control Number: 2009931316

ISBN-13: 978-1-4354-9769-6

ISBN-10: 1-4354-9769-4

Delmar
5 Maxwell Drive
Clifton Park, NY 12065–2919
USA

Cengage Learning products are represented in Canada by Nelson Education, Ltd.

For your lifelong learning solutions, visit **delmar.cengage.com**

Visit our corporate website at **www.cengage.com**

Notice to the Reader
Publisher does not warrant or guarantee any of the products described herein or perform any independent analysis in connection with any of the product information contained herein. Publisher does not assume, and expressly disclaims, any obligation to obtain and include information other than that provided to it by the manufacturer. The reader is expressly warned to consider and adopt all safety precautions that might be indicated by the activities described herein and to avoid all potential hazards. By following the instructions contained herein, the reader willingly assumes all risks in connection with such instructions. The publisher makes no representations or warranties of any kind, including but not limited to, the warranties of fitness for particular purpose or merchantability, nor are any such representations implied with respect to the material set forth herein, and the publisher takes no responsibility with respect to such material. The publisher shall not be liable for any special, consequential, or exemplary damages resulting, in whole or part, from the readers' use of, or reliance upon, this material.

Printed in Canada
1 2 3 4 5 6 13 12 11 10 9

*To my wife, my kids,
and my fine-feathered friends.*

CONTENTS

Preface   *vii*

Foreword   *ix*

CHAPTER 1   Science of Fear   1
CHAPTER 2   Churkendoose   5
CHAPTER 3   Locked-In   9
CHAPTER 4   Complex and Odd   13
CHAPTER 5   Super Models   17
CHAPTER 6   Strange Cures   21
CHAPTER 7   Compassion Fatigue   25
CHAPTER 8   Tingo   29
CHAPTER 9   Broca's Brain: Brother, Wherefore Art Thou?   33
CHAPTER 10   Cook and Kiwi   39
CHAPTER 11   Cell Hell   43
CHAPTER 12   Profanity   49
CHAPTER 13   X-Ray Eyes   53
CHAPTER 14   Mixed Metaphors   57
CHAPTER 15   The Lonely Whale   61
CHAPTER 16   Feral Children   65
CHAPTER 17   Biology of Hope   71
CHAPTER 18   Dreams   75
CHAPTER 19   A Little Night *Tafelspitz*   79
CHAPTER 20   Whales, Brains, and Islands   83
CHAPTER 21   Time After Time   87
CHAPTER 22   Moxon and the Flying Trapeze   91
CHAPTER 23   Sushi, Gator Tail, and Knee Banjos   95
CHAPTER 24   Snake Wine and Culture Shock   99
CHAPTER 25   Never Odd or Even   103

CHAPTER 26	The Sociology of Aphasia	107
CHAPTER 27	Proverbs	113
CHAPTER 28	Laugh Pills	117
CHAPTER 29	Sage Advice	121
CHAPTER 30	Holidays and Youth	125
CHAPTER 31	St. Anthony and Motor Speech	129
CHAPTER 32	Saguaros and Dogwoods: Change and Ethics	133
CHAPTER 33	Light in the Attic	137
CHAPTER 34	Morphology and the Red Priest	141
CHAPTER 35	Turn, Turn, Turn	145
CHAPTER 36	Dictionaries	149
CHAPTER 37	Cultures	153
CHAPTER 38	Aquarius	157
CHAPTER 39	Personal Accounts	161
CHAPTER 40	Bad Science — Good Science	165
CHAPTER 41	Eggheads	169
CHAPTER 42	Lives	173
CHAPTER 43	Days-Daze	177
CHAPTER 44	Rotten Reviews	181
CHAPTER 45	Mentors	185
CHAPTER 46	Quality	189
CHAPTER 47	Strikes	193
CHAPTER 48	Surf and Space	197
CHAPTER 49	On Being a Patient	201
CHAPTER 50	First Among Gifts	205
CHAPTER 51	Growth	209
CHAPTER 52	Classification	213
CHAPTER 53	Fruit Bats and Apples	217
CHAPTER 54	The Bran	221
CHAPTER 55	Voices	223
CHAPTER 56	The Grass	225
CHAPTER 57	Marching	227
CHAPTER 58	Term, Holidays, Work	229
CHAPTER 59	Brain and Red Rocks	231
CHAPTER 60	Crossing to Safety	233
CHAPTER 61	Objectives, Scope, Philosophy	237
Epilogue		243
Index		245

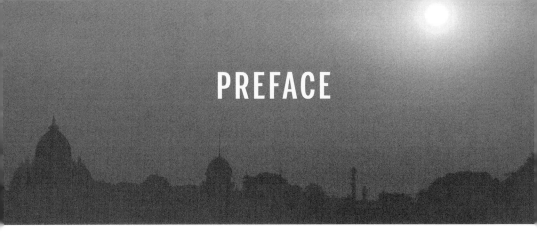

PREFACE

INTRODUCTION

The primary audience for this collection of essays on language, laughter, and life will be professionals, clinicians, and students in communication science and disorders. An important secondary audience would be professionals and students in English, Creative Writing, and Linguistics. This collection is quite eclectic in its topic spread and is appropriate for a wide audience of the educated public.

WHY I WROTE THIS COLLECTION

This is a collection of essays written as editorials to each quarterly issue of the *Journal of Medical Speech-Language Pathology*. Sixty-one essays have been selected from a span of 17 volumes of the journal. The topics are on a wide range of intellectually stimulating topics including essays on snake wine, profanity, and feral children. These essays were written to color a view of the world that values the importance of language, linguistic regularities and oddities, humor and laughter, and off-beat attention-grabbing topics.

ORGANIZATION OF THE TEXT

The collection of essays is organized in roughly reverse chronological order from the present to 1995.

FEATURES

This collection features brief essays on 61 different topics. The book could be used as examples of short story or essay writing to improve the literacy of students; interesting sideboard reading on life and language; or on values of scientific literacy and critical-analytical thinking.

ABOUT THE AUTHOR

Leonard L. "Chick" LaPointe, PhD is the Distinguished Professor of Communication Science and Disorders at Florida State University. He also holds appointments in the Program of Neuroscience and the College of Medicine at Florida State University. He is Co-Director of the Neurolinguistic-Neurocognitive Research Center at Tallahassee Memorial Hospital and founding Editor-in-Chief of the *Journal of Medical Speech-Language Pathology*. Dr. LaPointe has written 5 books, over 40 book chapters, and over 80 journal articles on brain-based disorders of human communication and cognition. He has held visiting research professorships at the University of Queensland, Australia; the University of Hong Kong; and the University of Canterbury in Christchurch, New Zealand. He has presented over 400 papers and lectures throughout the world from Singapore to Brazil and has been honored by distinguished alumni awards from Michigan State University and the University of Colorado.

ACKNOWLEDGMENTS

I wish to acknowledge Dr. Sadanand Singh and Angie Singh of Plural Publishing, Inc. The Singhs created the *Journal of Medical Speech-Language Pathology* nearly 20 years ago when it was born of a Singular mother. They always encouraged me to "express yourself" in the essays and that has been a most therapeutic endeavor. I would like to thank Sherry Dickinson of Delmar, Cengage Learning who made this happen. I also would like to acknowledge the support of my lovely, respected, and completely other-oriented wife, who makes Mother Teresa seem indifferent.

—Leonard L. LaPointe, PhD

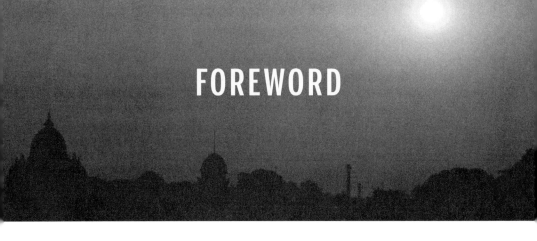

FOREWORD

There is an effortless reverence among the intelligent for language mastery.

—Jim Harrison (2002)

Leonard (Chick) LaPointe's brother and sisters never found a book in the Channing, Michigan, library he had not previously checked out. Don't let the nickname fool you, he was not a callow youth. The boy was a reader; the man is a reader—and writer. Cengage Learning is publishing *Journal of Medical Speech-Language Pathology: Voices: Collected Essays on Language, Laughter, and Life,* a collection of Chick's editorials written to introduce nearly every number of the *Journal of Medical Speech-Language Pathology* since he willed that journal into existence in March 1993. The publisher asked me for a foreword. My effortless reverence for Chick's language mastery made acceptance easy.

His first essay, *Objectives, Scope, Philosophy* was a harbinger. He wanted the journal to be a conduit "that facilitates the creation of knowledge and the birth of ideas," an archive "for a growing clinical science," and a wellspring of suggestions and direction for clinicians. Progress toward these objectives was evident from the first volume. The scope was to be unrestricted. Because disease is indifferent to age and because medically oriented speech-language pathologists offer cradle to grave services, Chick decided:

"We will not restrict our focus to any segment of the life span." Because clinicians were increasingly busy with a sometimes bewildering assortment of medical and cognitive, linguistic, and motor, including swallowing disorders, he equally welcomed papers on the most and least common. Because clinicians are often punished for unbillable hours spent reading, he wanted the articles to be trustworthy so that clinicians would not need to spend extra time checking veracity. As editor, he wanted to bring "tact, diplomacy, good judgment, appropriate humor, and professionalism." Readers and contributors know how well he and his journal have lived up to these dignified aims.

Had his and his journal's contributions to clinical science and practice stopped there, the profession would have been well-served. Chick, however, had more in mind. This lover of words, metaphors, puns, palindromes, scatology, alliteration, rhyme, synecdoche, proverbs, legerdemain, and anaphora (and hater of cell phone abuse, fear mongering, and indifference to the human condition) began introducing each number of the journal with an essay. They went unlabeled until 2001 and were called editorials thereafter. From first to last, these essays have been personal, funny, and unexpected. Who knew an editor would allow readers to see behind the words—his and those of his contributors? Who knew one's appetite for impersonal scientific writing could be whetted by essays so personal that reading them sometimes seemed like innocent voyeurism?

From the beginning he showed the prescience that would become one of his hallmarks. He correctly predicted that serious clinical scientists with something to say wanted evidence of this new journal's viability before they said it in JMS-LP. Seventeen years later that evidence is undeniable, but even early on it was clear that Chick would accept nothing else. Even in Volume I, Number 1, the journal's contributions to clinical science were clear. Equally clear was Chick's firm, humane, and intellectual guidance of the journal's development. The essay introducing Volume I, Number 2 expressed his hope that the contents would "provoke thought, understanding and perhaps enlighten the path of clinical management." It did as have all the other numbers of all the other volumes. I'm just one of many who sees even the most treacherous clinical path more clearly because of something I read in the journal. And so the tone was set for the journal and for the essays.

Wallace Stegner, whose novel, *Crossing to Safety*, probably gave Chick that first essay's title, would have appreciated it and all those that followed. And he would not have been surprised at Chick's and the journal's success and durability. Instead he would have recognized Chick as a compatriot. Stegner, when asked how he managed to create a bookshelf of writings and to meet deadlines year after year, said of his talent "It's like a beaver's teeth . . . you keep doing it because that's really what you're made to do, that's what you want to do." And so, however inelegant the metaphor, Chick, too, has continued to chew away. (My apologies Chick, if at a roast in some, we hope, distant time, someone shows up in prosthetic buck teeth and makes splashing sounds in a bowl of water.)

Reading these 61 essays in three settings as I did is like hovering over a landscape. Patterns emerge. Chick loves language and its restoration. Read *Complex and Odd*: "Language is such a complexity. Intricate, only partially rule-governed; fraught with linguistic pot holes that can knock off a tongue-wheel or derail a perfectly inferred meaning." He mourns those whose language, speech, or voice is disrupted by disease. Read *Voices*: "Sometimes voices love their sweetness. Sometimes the joy turns to anguish when sweet voice is lost." He rejoices in those of us who work to restore language, speech, or voice. Read *The Lonely Whale*: ". . . our mission is indispensable. We get up in the morning so we can help all those who are at risk for isolation and unwanted solitude. We yearn to help them communicate with the pod," or *Locked In*: "Each day, in some way, we help replace the butterflies." He values science and abhors pseudo science. Read *X-Ray Eyes*: "Scientific literacy seems to be waging an uphill battle against the spewing of sensationalism, reductionism, and bad science that fills our airwaves and sells tabloids." Third graders provide some of his most compelling peeks into language (and spelling). Read *Eggheads*: "Thank you for the very fun and faceanayeding time here at Cerritos. The front of the brain looks like Elvis's hare." A youngster who understands s's may well have meant hare. And why waste a perfectly good "i" when bran works just fine as an alternate spelling for brain?

He promised JMS-LP would be international. It has been and so has he. Paris (*Broca's Brain: Brother Wherefore Art Thou?*). Vienna (*A Little Night Tafelspitz*). New Zealand (*Cook and Kiwi*). Hong Kong (*Snake Wine and Culture Shock*). Venice (*Morphology and the Red Priest*). Australia (*Fruit Bats and Apples*).

He recognized that one's view is best while being held aloft by one's teachers. Thus he has praised his and the profession's progenitors in essays such as *Mentors* and *Growth*. For him it was Mrs. Kurth, Dr. Ned Welcome Bowler, and Dr. Robert Terrence Wertz. Mrs. Kurth set him on the road to learning. Bowler and Wertz kept him from drifting across the centerline. For the profession it was Ray Kent who paved the way. Innumerable other colleagues receive his praise as part of his introduction to their journal contributions. No other journal makes its contributors feel quite so much a part of an intellectual community.

He uses biography to remind us about professional humility. What better reminder that even the best of us usually end up tied for first place than his essay: *Moxon and the Flying Trapeze*? Moxon was Broca's (*Lives*) contemporary.

Professional citizenship has always been one of Chick's priorities. Thus descriptions of meetings and meeting sites appear regularly in this group of essays. His description of San Antonio (Yangaguana or refreshing waters to Native Americans) and the Motor Speech and Motor Speech Disorders Conference is typical. "San Antonio was an appropriate setting for the pursuit and dissemination of the latest neuroscientific and clinical information on understanding and restoring lost speech" because after all St. Anthony is the Saint of lost things, and what causes a greater sense of loss than impaired communication? After reading this essay, readers will be sorry they missed the meeting, if they did, and those who attended that conference will wonder how they missed so much. He does the same for the Clinical Aphasiology Conferences in Sedona (*Brain and Red Rocks*), Montana (*Days Daze*), and Orca Island (*Whales, Brains, and Islands*).

One of Chick's greatest virtues is his advocacy for the men, women, and children with communication problems. He reminds us that spirit is not lost when language is (*Strokes*). He reminds us that treatment of speech, voice, or language succeeds only if the person rather than the disorder is treated. He reminds us that humanity rather than political correctness is the reason for person-first language: not aphasia but person with aphasia (*On Being a Patient*; *The Sociology of Aphasia*). He saves some of his highest praise for those organizations such as the National Aphasia Association devoted to people with communication problems (*Light in the Attic*).

Language mastery is evident on every page. Chick's prose is by turns picaresque, joyful, adventurous, teasing, antic, risky, and just plain damn good. Clearly Chick loves words (and syntax). His essay *Never Odd Or Even* could not have been Never Odd Nor Even. Who knew the Inuit word for "To exchange wives for a few days only" was "aredjarekput?" Or that Luida and Roger Flavell published *Dictionary of Proverbs and Their Origins* in 1996, or at all? Or what the T word is in George Carlin's list of seven words (S, P, F, C, C, M, and T) you couldn't say on TV? Or that Dan Rather may have said, "Frankly, we don't know whether to wind the watch or bark at the moon?" In these essays a period may mark the edge of a cliff, the fringe of a magic carpet, or the chair concealing a whoopee cushion.

These essays make me strive. They make me look up and out. They make me laugh and rewrite even simple sentences half a dozen times. They make me even more proud of what I do. Enough. Discover or rediscover for yourself. I'll send a copy to Jim Harrison.

REFERENCES

Etulain, R.W., and Wallace Stegner, Western Humanist. In C.E. Rankin (Ed.). *Wallace Stegner: Man and Writer*. Albuquerque: University of New Mexico Press. 1996, pp. 49–60.

Harrison, Jim. *Off to the Side*. New York: Atlantic Monthly Press. 2002.

CHAPTER 1

SCIENCE OF FEAR

Fear grows in darkness; if you think there's a bogeyman around, turn on the light.

—Dorothy Thompson

If you think there is a monster in your closet or a shark in your bathtub turn on the light; both literally and figuratively. As the cartoon chicken said, "I have a morbid fear of heavy luggage. I'm carrying around a lot of baggage." Most of us carry this baggage around day and night; especially at night. Some fear is good. It protects us and it is rationale. A lot of fear is not so good. It creates a phobic, anxiety-ridden existence that prevents us from smelling the caramel macchiato and drives us nuts. A recent book by a Canadian journalist, Daniel Gardner attempts to put fear in perspective. *The Science of Fear* (Gardner, 2008) is getting a lot of air time and attention and tackles a topic that defies our amygdaloid-infused inflammatory belief systems and tosses a healthy dose of cool reason on miscalculated risk and fear. Gardner's book is full of the latest interpretations of neuroscience and attempts to balance the struggle between our emotional-reptilian-survival brain and our rationale, thinking, neocortex. He says a lot of what humans fear springs from how humans miscalculate risks. This constant tussle between what Gardner characterizes as "gut" (old brain) and "head" (new brain) does not always slant to the corner of reason and logic. It seems to be a lot easier to accept seditious fear than to be calmed by probability and statistics. These gut-based fears are reddened and escalated by ubiquitous societal fear mongering. Politicians use it. The media lives by it ("if it bleeds it's on page one"). Corporations and special interest groups fatten their revenue with it. It's everywhere. It's everywhere. Think of a few trailers you've heard for news telecasts. *"Can a common virus make you fat?" "Starbucks pulls peanut butter products." "Baby bottles may cause early puberty." "Pack of wild cocker spaniels terrorizes Wyoming."* We are inundated with these scare headlines everyday and not just from the tabloid press. The information tsunami that we experience increasingly with our digital ever-connected access through the Internet and cell phones insures that we have warnings and scare stories bombarding us from all the directions of our GPS day and night. This, as Gardner and company indicate, insures that not only are we never not at work, but that we are showered with miscalculated risk scare stories that cause needless worry. Paul Slovic, a University of Oregon psychology professor and former president of The Society for Risk Analysis says on Gardner's dustcover "Those of us who spend our careers in research hope that someone like Daniel Gardner will come along and bring our findings to the world in an engaging and scientifically accurate way."

Gardner cites a lot of respectable examples in his book, including bunches of scare headlines that are caused by "denominator blindness." The media routinely tell us the number of people that are maimed or killed by some new threat, but rarely inform us of the denominator (out of how many people). He cites an article from *The Times* of London. The newspaper reported that the number of Britons murdered by strangers had "increased by a third in eight years." The total had increased from 99 to 130. But the article failed to mention the denominator, that there are approximately 60 million Britons, so the chance of being murdered by a stranger increased from 99 in 60 million to 130 in 60 million. As they say, do the math, and discover that the risk has risen from an almost invisible 0.0001 percent to an almost invisible 0.00015 percent. There should be far more worry about the very real health risks from automobile accidents and diabetes. These same miscalculated risks have influenced our undue concern over West Nile virus, terrorism, salmonella from tomatoes, and air travel. Gardner attempts to put all of these risks that have been carefully nurtured by systems of fear mongering into manageable perspective.

Some fears are indeed rationale. It is rational to fear drivers who are yakking away on their cell phones while eating or applying makeup. But many fears are irrational. We all harbor some irrational tidbits that we know make no logical sense, but nevertheless kick start our limbic and autonomic nervous systems. These irrational fears are the breeding ground of anxiety disorders and panic attacks. But some are difficult to reconcile. A cruise through the Internet reveals some interesting and amusing sites devoted to irrational fears. In fact one blog entitled *Irrational Fears* http://theonlythingtofearisfearitself .blogspot.com/ cites quite a list:

- I'm terrified of Abraham Lincoln.
- Spontaneous combustion
- Pictures of whale's tails . . . I imagine me in a kayak
- Butterflies
- Bathtub sharks
- Windmills
- Rainbows. The larger and more vibrant they are, the more horrible in my opinion. Sometimes I scream when a rainbow catches me off-guard.
- Hawaii
- Pickles
- That someone will throw a lit cigarette out of their moving car onto the street and when I drive over it, it could somehow blow up my car. (I have to admit to this one myself.)
- Being hunted for sport
- Dogs ears being turned inside out
- The serrated metal edge on boxes of plastic wrap
- Leprechauns, clowns, ventriloquist dummies, and Santa Claus
- People who've had too much Botox® and other expressionless mannequins
- Every time I sit down on the toilet, I'm pretty sure that a large sewer rat will have somehow made its way through the pipes.

Well, there is some fodder for the expansion of your own special list of irrational fears. I'm sorry if I've implanted some of these, and if you will now have to start checking the bathtub for sharks and avoiding rainbows. Miscalculated risk can be a serious source of unnecessary fear. Daniel Gardner alerts us to this danger and presents a readable and scientifically-based report on the topic.

As the underappreciated and eminent woman journalist Dorothy Thompson recommended, just turn on the light (Kurth, 1990).

REFERENCES

Gardner, D. (2008). *The science of fear.* New York: Penguin Group. *Irrational fears.* Retrieved January 27, 2009 from http://theonlythingtofearisfearitself .blogspot.com/

Kurth, P. (1990). *American Cassandra: The life of Dorothy Thompson.* Boston: Little, Brown.

CHAPTER 2

CHURKENDOOSE

It depends on how you look at things . . .

—Ray Bolger (1947)

Once upon a time, in a land of icicles and rabbits, not too far from the shores of Lake Superior, lived a few hardy people who scratched away in the mines and forests and on the railroads in a sometimes zero-sum attempt to make a living. The children of these scrappers and scramblers knew no other world except what Mrs. Kurth taught them about Baffin Island and the Belgian Congo. They attended little brick or wooden schools, sometimes with all 12 grades in the same building, and they welcomed and celebrated the seasons (fishing, hunting, trapping, berry, potato, baseball, basketball, spring, summer, partridge, deer, ski-jumping, winter, winter, and winter). In that setting my sister Sally and I, (and maybe a few of our siblings, though we were separated in birth order by eons), spent a lot of those winter days building ice forts and then retreating to our grandmother's console record player when the first signs of purple-green frost-bitten fingers began to appear. That's where we met the Churkendoose. This old Decca 78 rpm kiddy folk opera was played until it smoked, and we sang along with Ray Bolger (already a star from his classic role as the Scarecrow in *The Wizard of Oz*), and perhaps learned some of the lessons of empathy, inclusion, and tolerance articulated in classic Churkendoose fashion by classic philosophers such as Martin Buber.

The Churkendoose in text form was written in 1946 by Ben Ross Berenberg with pictures by Dellwyn Cunningham and published as a Wonder Book by a Division of Grosset & Dunlap in New York. Somehow it, and its Ray Bolger interpreted recording, reached the hamlets of Upper Michigan and we loved it. The message was thinly veiled, important, and as relevant today as it was in the early 1950s. In fact it is echoed and reverberates in the recent political scene of the United States. In the original story as recorded in Bolger's wonderful Dorchester, Massachusetts dialect (he was the son of Portuguese and Irish parents), the Churkendoose tale champions the cause of misfits and teaches that beauty, compassion, and tolerance are in the eyes of the beholder. The Churkendoose just didn't fit in. He was part chicken, turkey, duck and goose. Churkendoose. The farm animals were dubious and skeptical and wanted to banish him. He was rejected and ridiculed. He talked in rhyme and danced instead of walked. And his message, as interpreted by Bolger, was classic:

It depends on how you look at things.
It depends on how you look at things.
Are the hippopotami, any handsomer than I?
Well it depends upon, begins and ends upon,
It all depends on how you look at things.

The Churkendoose eventually saves the other farm animals from the dreaded fox (who took off so fast it took three days for his shadow to catch up to him). The cheers arose from the farmyard and the farm fowl gathered around their hero in gratitude. He would have nothing of their hero worship. He just wanted to fit in and be accepted, as the rooster finally put it, "just because you're you." Finally, his differences were accepted and he was embraced by the farm society with genuineness. To listen to the opera and classical music composer Alec Wilder's composition and Ray Bolger's characterization of the Churkendoose try http://www.fluctu8.com/media/29180/4610/

It turns out that the lessons of the Churkendoose are eternal and elaborated upon by some the foremost philosophers of contemporary thinking. As Randy Best of the North Carolina Center for Ethics puts it, the central message of this tale is that preconceptions, even long existing rules about the way things are to work, should never be allowed to limit the value of another in our eyes. The Churkendoose Story celebrates tolerance and diversity. As Best states, we strive to make a human connection with others and to experience empathy, sympathy and compassion in our daily human connections.

Martin Buber, the philosopher, scholar and social activist, identified such a connection in his philosophy of Dialogue, described in his work, *Ich und Du,* translated as I and Thou. *Ich-Du* ("I-Thou" or "I-You") is a relationship that stresses the mutual, holistic existence of two beings. It is a singular relationship because these beings meet one another and exist without any qualification or objectification of one another. Buber's ideas are far reaching and even extend to the thorny political and historic problems of the Middle East. Buber's philosophy describes a desire to live in peace and brotherhood with a common homeland and the development of a republic in which all peoples have the possibility of free development. Buber rejected the idea of nationalistic special interests as just another divisive political movement and wanted instead to see the creation of an exemplary society.

How great the leap from the barnyard to the globe. Where is the Churkendoose when we need him? The lessons of Mr. Rogers, Rudolph the Red-Nosed Reindeer, Martin Buber, and the Churkendoose are blended into an unseemly and timeless pastiche. Yet how close and elementary these lessons may be. Perhaps the Churkendoose is worth digging up again. Is a baby chimpanzee, any uglier than me? Well it depends on how you look at things.

REFERENCES

Best, R. (2002). Platform talk delivered to the North Carolina Society for Ethical Culture. Retrieved November 2, 2008 from http://www.ncethicalsociety.org/rb.empathy.d090802.shtml

Buber, M. (2006). *I and Thou,* translated by Ronald Gregor Smith. New York: Charles Scribner's Sons, 1958.

Bolger, R., as *The Churkendoose.* (1947). Story and Words by Ben Ross Berenberg; Music by Alec Wilder, Decca CU 103.

Wilder, Alec. Retrieved November 2, 2008 from http://www.fluctu8.com/media/29180/4610/

CHAPTER 3

LOCKED-IN

*The identity badge pinned to Sandrine's white tunic says
'Speech Therapist,' but it should read 'Guardian Angel.'*

—Jean-Dominique Bauby (1997)

Locked-in syndrome is a rare neurological disorder characterized by complete or nearly complete paralysis of voluntary muscles in all parts of the body except for those of muscles of the upper face and those that control eye movement. It may result from riding a motorcycle into a bridge abutment, a drunken dive from a Mexican balcony during spring break, nasty diseases that destroy the fatty, myelin sheath surrounding nerve fibers, from an overdose of poisons or medicine, or from a deep-brain stroke. It should not be wished on the worst of enemies. It leaves the unfortunate few (or maybe not so few) who experience it unable to move and unable to speak. Completely mute and paralyzed. People who are locked-in are fully conscious and can think, reason, imagine, dream, and have full tacit command of the language system they learned. But they cannot move or speak. At this point in neurologic history there is no cure; nor much of a standard course of treatment. Treatment is symptomatic and supportive, and many survivors with locked-in syndrome have a reduced life expectancy barring other medical complications, but 10 year survival rates as high as 80% have been reported. Mostly, locked-in syndrome is caused by damage to the ventral pons of the brainstem, that pear-shaped knob that is filled with transverse and up-and-down fiber tracts that relay movement and sensory signals between and among the cerebellum, cerebrum, and other subcortical structures. It is a knob of great consequence, perhaps secondary only to a few other knobs of the body, and when it is greatly damaged we die. If it is partially damaged, we may be left locked-in. Some would contend there is no difference. This horrific neuropathology has come to the consciousness of the general public at least a couple of times in the last decade. Jean-Dominique Bauby is chiefly responsible for both of these peaks of awareness of being locked-in. Bauby was a 42 year-old father of two and Editor-in-Chief of *Elle,* the ultra-chic fashion magazine in Paris. While driving with his son, he suffered a massive stroke which left him locked-in. After a period of coma, he awakened and was transferred to a seaside hospital in France and that is where he met his "Guardian Angel," Sandrine. She was as they call it in France, an *orthophoniste*, or speech-language pathologist (or speech therapist or phono-audiologist or communication disorders specialist, or speech clinician, or a dozen other ambiguous and poorly-understood appellations that have hindered awareness and understanding of our profession for generations). Bauby had been unable to communicate beyond rudimentary signals and was trapped in what he regarded as his "diving bell."

Along came Sandrine and discovered that Jean-Do, as his friends called him, could blink his left eye. She promptly took advantage of this kernel of a remaining movement and instructed Bauby to blink his eye when he heard her say the French letter that she named in sequence. She wrote it down and he was able to make a word. Then words. Then sentences. Then release the "butterflies" of his imagination, thoughts, and emotions and finally, finally, communication. In fact, with the guidance of Sandrine and another young woman, Claude, he eventually wrote his nearly 140 page memoir, entitled *The Diving Bell and the Butterfly* (1997). I read this book shortly after its publication and in fact wrote a review of it for this Journal that appeared in the

March, 1998 issue. In it I pointed out that the small book was much more than an inspirational study of courage and triumph of the human spirit. I noted Bauby's caustic wit, some bitterness, understandable anger, and a fine and literate sense of metaphor, and sarcasm. One particularly evocative chapter was called Through a Glass Darkly. Through his tedious letter-by-letter dictation Bauby communicated the poignancy of a visit by his children. He was wheeled to a patch of sand dune open to the sun and the sea and played Hangman with his son while watching his daughter Celeste do cartwheels in the sand. He ruminated about the personalities and future of his children, as all of us are wont to do. Finally, in Jean-Do's words, "They have left. The car will already be speeding toward Paris. I sink into contemplation of a drawing by Celeste, which we immediately pinned to the wall: a kind of two-headed fish with blue-lashed eyes and multicolored scales. But what is interesting in the drawing is its oval shape, which bears a disconcerting resemblance to the mathematical symbol for infinity."

Jean-Dominique Bauby died of cardiac failure two days after his book was published in Paris. Despite the tragedy inherent in Jean-Do's story and life, Bauby has left something wondrous behind. The second wave of Bauby's story has been realized by the release of the remarkable film adaptation of his book by director Julian Schnabel. I've seen it twice now; the second screening at our local Student Life building here at Florida State University that allowed me to participate in a panel discussion after the film screening. The empathy and effect of the film on the audience was remarkable. Most of the good books we like are disappointing as a film, but not this one. Schnabel is first an artist, and he has created a remarkable and award-winning celluloid treatment of Jean-Do's book. Breathtaking visuals and dynamic performances make this a powerful capture of Jean-Dominique's locked-in syndrome and of his remarkable spirit that has allowed the butterflies of empathy, emotion, imagination, and the richness of human communication to escape the diving bell of locked-in syndrome. This is a story that should be on our shelves in both its extraordinary written and film form. It is particularly relevant to those of us who toil in the vineyards of the restoration of communication. In the blinked-out words of Jean-Dominique Bauby, "speech therapy is an art that deserves to be more widely known." Each day, in some way, we help release the butterflies.

REFERENCES

Bauby, Jean-Dominique (1997). *The diving bell and the butterfly*. New York: Alfred A Knopf.

LaPointe, L. L. (1998). The diving bell and the butterfly: (*Le Scaphandre et Le Papillon*). *Journal of Medical Speech-Language Pathology*, 6, 1, 51–52.

CHAPTER 4

COMPLEX AND ODD

Language is the mother, not the handmaiden of thought;
words will tell you things you never thought or felt before.

—W. H. Auden (1990)

How do we ever learn it? Language is such a complexity. Intricate; only partially rule-governed; fraught with linguistic potholes that can knock off a tongue-wheel or derail a perfectly inferred meaning. No wonder there are marvelous professional fields that have evolved to help fix it. It is so complex. *Complexity* is the term often used to characterize something with many parts in intricate arrangement. In information processing, complexity is a degree of the total number of properties transmitted by an object and discerned by an observer. Such a collection of properties is often referred to as a *state*. I thought Michigan was a state. And Upper Michigan was a sovereign nation. Scientists and the rest of us are perpetually awash in complexity, and many scientific disciplines devote their sweating, waking hours dealing with complex states, systems, and phenomena. Indeed, some would say that only bits and pieces that are complex are truly elegant, interesting and worthy of study. Perhaps these are the specialists and scientists who fall into the rabbit hole of string theory and chaos theory and other attempts to organize randomness. Some fields have had to develop their own specific definitions of complexity, and there is a more recent movement to regroup observations from different fields to study *complexity* in itself, whether it appears in honeybee colonies, human brains, or football fantasy team exercises. One such interdisciplinary effort that appears to be budding is characterized as the study of *relational order theories*.

Well, we have our own complexity in the wondrous world of language. Lemmas beget phonemes, beget morphemes beget syllables, beget words, beget spreading activation, beget some semblance of predictability, beget perhaps a shred of meaning. Mostly. Most of the time. Sometimes never. Language is so complex and brilliant when it works. Yet the evolution of languages has not prevented nor naturally selected out the implicit lingui-trapdoors that trick us and trap us ever so frequently. Sometimes we have to scratch our heads (our collective head or singularly for those of us with two).

George Carlin the pundit and comedian has made a good living by observing and pointing out the complexities of language and how odd it can be. Yet we learn it and use it and sometimes do not even pause to consider the oddities inherent in our use of this marvelous gift. Consider the following Carlinesque examples:

- How can a slim chance and a fat chance be the same?
- After a number of lidocaine injections, my jaw got number.
- A bass was painted on the head of the bass drum.
- Exactly what is so fast about quicksand?
- The farm was used to produce produce.
- The buck does strange things when the does are around.
- It's fruitless to eat vegetables.
- She wound a bandage around the wound.
- You can set a broken bone; you can set hair after you shampoo it; you can set a poem to music; set sail; or sit in front of your television set while a jelly sets in the fridge.

So how is it that amid such complexity little ones learn language so readily? For most adults, the struggles and trials of acquisition are only a distant memory. We have learned to deal with our language both functionally and in some cases evocatively despite its quirkiness and ambiguity and do not think twice about it until for some reason it becomes scrambled or lost. When someone upsets the intracranial scrabble board, language loss comes to new levels of awareness. Those of us who have worked with disjointed communication have no doubt heard the sentiment echoed repeatedly, as one of my clients with aphasia said, "I took it all for granted. You never miss the water till the smell goes dry. I thought I was beginning to lose my table."

Enjoy the oddities and the occasional regularity and predictability of this complex mother, language. Auden surely did. And if you want to continue to have fun despite the complexity, try *Wordplay: A Curious Dictionary of Language Oddities* by Chris Cole.

REFERENCES

Auden, W. H. (1990). *Forewords and afterwords.* New York: Vintage.

Cole, C. (1999). *Wordplay: A curious dictionary of language oddities.* New York: Sterling Publishing Co.

CHAPTER 5

SUPER MODELS

To tell a woman everything she may not do is to tell her what she can do.

—Spanish Proverb

Speech-language pathology is overwhelmingly a profession of females. Males currently comprise 4.4% of speech-language pathologists (SLPs). Few professions are nearly 96% female. Overall, the proportion of male American Speech-Language-Hearing (ASHA) constituents has declined steadily from 8.3% in 1997 to 7.7% in 1999, 7.2% in 2001, 6.7% in 2003, 6.3% in 2005, and 6.2% at year end 2006 (Demographics, ASHA website, 2007). What this trend will eventually mean for the profession remains to be seen, and ASHA has been working for several years to address the effects of this gender inequity on remuneration, prestige, and the scientific basis of the discipline.

At first thought, some might conclude that choosing a female-dominated profession would be the ideal solution for a woman within what is perceived by some as an oppressing male-dominated workforce. Some may view this choice as relief from the power struggle for recognition and promotion within a context of greater competition. These gossamer illusions of relief are not real. To some, these are basic assumptions that tail along with all of the other misguided presumptions and stereotypes about women in the workforce. What may have been created, however, is a tide on which all boats rise or descend. Pay inequity, unrewarded administrative power, and double duty across domestic and work responsibilities are alive and well, even in female dominated professions. These issues exist as well within the added societal reality of lower prestige for the female professions. Low prestige is an attribute of nearly all of these (Freidl, 1995; Turner, 2007). Nurses, teachers, childcare workers, librarians, secretaries, and toenail painters all deal with condescension and inadequate remuneration compared to their testosterone-infused counterparts.

Surely much of the problem is societal. The view and worth of women across societies or cultures varies greatly, and one does not have to stray too far from the stories in the daily newspaper to see examples of crude and cruel gender discrimination. One particularly dramatic report was an observation by a Western reporter. When he inquired if times and attitudes had changed about the status of women in a particular war-torn country because he noticed women now walked ahead of men on country roads, whereas before they always trailed several steps behind men, the response was "there are still lots of mines unexploded."

A minefield of another nature is the influence of advertising and media on the image of females in Western societies. The visual aspects of the media influence young females early and may be a factor in perceptions of self-worth, eating disorders, and choice of profession. We are inundated with tens of thousands of messages each week that "young and thin and pretty" is good and "old or fat or plain-looking" is bad. Sexist and ageist advertising is a way of life in most industrialized cultures, and it is no surprise that it inculcates these values and mores into developing minds. People in advertisements rarely look like ordinary people. Because models are selling a product, advertisers use computer technology to erase models' "flaws" because they believe it will make their product more appealing. In the past few decades, the media's standard of perfection has grown increasingly unhealthy and unrealistic. Twenty years ago, models weighed 8% less than the average woman; today they weigh 23% less (Children's Media Project, 2007). According to some sources, 90% of

American girls aged 3–11 own Barbie dolls and live in a world with a fairy tale princess as their role model. Could anyone be unaware of the underlying messages that these figures contain?

So it is refreshing when along comes a genuinely healthy role model for females in the professions; a model that emphasizes achievement, intelligence, and skills rather than carefully sculpted, buffed, painted, and surgically enhanced body parts. Good role models abound in our female dominated profession, and they exist as well in traditionally male bastions.

Katrina Firlik is a neurosurgeon, one of only 200 or so women who labor daily among the alpha males who run the packs in this high-pressure, ultra-prestige medical specialty. She is also a talented writer, and one of her latest offerings is titled *Another Day in the Frontal Lobe: A Brain Surgeon Exposes Life on the Inside* (Firlik, 2006). She writes about her influences; about acceptance; the tools and risks and emotions of her profession; and about the daily inundation of patients who need to come to grips with the less than glamorous problems involved in an aging spine.

One of the many invigorating parts of Firlik's book is the obvious respect she has for other neuroscientists, and not just those at the perceived top of the pecking order who ablate and repair brain tissue. She expresses deep reverence for Ph.D. professionals with whom she has worked, such as Marcel Just and Pat Carpenter at Carnegie-Mellon University who have distinguished careers in the study of speech, comprehension, visual-spatial skills, memory, and decision making. The complexity of this nether land of higher level cognition and mental abilities does not escape her, and she gives ample regard to those of us who toil in those bleak and sometimes veiled fields of neuroscience.

Katrina Firlik's work is worth reading. It is genuinely well written, and it has a not so occult message that women can compete on any level and in any discipline. She is indeed a super role model and no doubt will provide inspiration as well as a reality check to younger women contemplating a professional life. As Maya Angelou might say, we need more heroes and she-roes.

REFERENCES

Demographics. ASHA website. Retrieved October 14, 2007, from http://www.asha.org/about/membership-certification/member-counts.htm

Children's media project. Images of women in the media. Retrieved October 15, 2007, from http://www.childrensmediaproject.org/article.asp?showid=47

Firlik, K. (2006). *Another day in the frontal lobe: A brain surgeon exposes life on the inside*. New York: Random House.

Friedl, E. (1995). The life of an academic: A personal record of a teacher, administrator, and anthropologist. *Annual Review of Anthropology*, 24, 1–19.

Turner, B. (2007). A female-dominated profession in the male-dominated workforce of higher education: Set against the backdrop of *The handmaid's tale*. Retrieved October 14, 2007, from http://www.fsu.edu/helps/hardee/paperssummer02/turner.pdf

CHAPTER 6

STRANGE CURES

Doctors are men who prescribe medicines of which they know little, to cure diseases of which they know less, in human beings of whom they know nothing.

— Voltaire

Have you ever wondered how to cure a hair ball? Well apparently it's petroleum jelly.

To prevent troublesome hair balls in your cat, apply a dollop of petroleum jelly to your cat's nose. The cat will lick off the jelly, lubricating any hair in its stomach so it can pass easily through the digestive system.

— http://www.stat.uga.edu/~molly/remedy.html

Recently while knocking around the Internet looking for some material on ancient approaches for treating stroke and aphasia, I happened on another of those fascinating and glue-like sites designed to make one fritter away 2 or 3 hours of time that could be more profitably spent on unraveling the secrets of time travel. That's where I stumbled onto the hair ball cure. I also discovered that dreaded toenail fungus can be cured by soaking your toes in mouthwash. Apparently, the powerful antiseptic leaves your toes looking healthy again and you certainly cannot deny the pleasure of getting a gentle waft of mint when you remove your socks. All of this directed me to a more authoritative source of information on ancient and contemporary cures titled, *Weird cures: The most hilarious, disgusting, and downright dangerous medical treatments ever!,* a quirky little paperback by Shram and Salmans (2006). These authors, who have an interesting bibliography including a book on slips of the tongue that derailed high-powered careers, have assembled a strange compilation of treatments and cures for nearly everything that has disgruntled humankind.

It occurred to me, as I continued my most enjoyable adventure on ancient and current day cures, that some of our contemporary thinking has not changed much since ancient times when it comes to treating much of the untreatable. The entire range of complimentary and alternative medicine (CAM), which until quite recently has not been burdened by the demands of empiricism, has been a historic mix of cures that surprisingly in many cases are well-founded and many more that are based solely on belief systems, exploitation, and scams.

Natural and homeopathic remedies abound that have turned out to be steeped in good science (think of the medicinal benefits of chocolate and wine for example and the advances in the diagnosis of diabetes by the observation that ants congregated on sugar-sweetened urine spots on the ground), but so many more have been based solely on testimonials and the drive to sell dubious and unregulated products. The *Skeptical Inquirer* and the Center for Skeptical Inquiry (http://www.csicop.org/) are sound sources for evaluating and debunking thinly veiled health claims and cures, and the cautious and critical thinker can do no better than to consult these sources regularly for intelligent and unbiased evaluation of cures.

With all of that in mind, and with the firm admonition to not try any of this at home without the consultation of a competent health care professional, we present a few of the weird, wonderful, and interesting remedies of both ancient and contemporary times garnered from a variety of sources. See if you can guess which is which.

- Smart splinter remover: Simply pour a drop of household glue all over the splinter, let dry, and peel the dried glue off the skin. The splinter sticks to the dried glue.
- Sleep apnea: Play the didgeridoo. First you have to find out what a didgeridoo is, then learn circular breathing, then learn to play the melodious moaning of this indigenous instrument from Australia. Our

frequent contributors from the University of Queensland can help you with this one. I'm not sure whether it is recommended that you play the indigenous didgeridoo in bed.

- Apoplexy (stroke): Apoplexy happens merely in the fleshy or overweight, and persons of disgusting or elevated livelihood. Action hoist the skull to an almost standing place; untie all tight clothing, thread, and relate chilly irrigate to the cranium and temperate irrigate to the bottom.

- Cleansing wounds: Larval therapy is effective as a debridement of wounds though has suffered historically from patient intolerance since many find the presence of maggots on their wounds to be socially inhibiting.

- Oatmeal for arthritis: Make a paste from cooked and slightly cooled oatmeal and apply to the hands for relief of arthritis pain. This may explain why I have sometimes noticed my friend Jay Rosenbek with his hands in his oatmeal bowl at breakfast.

- Bad breath: A Talmudic concoction to counteract offensive oral vapors is composed of dough water, olive oil, and salt. Another is the admonition to hold a pepper between the teeth.

- Eye puffiness: The shark oil in a popular commercially available hemorrhoidal ointment apparently contains a vasoconstrictor that can reduce swelling. The admonition is to avoid getting it in the eyes.

This last remedy was actually revealed in a videotaped interview with a graduate student and the late and great Dr. Jim Case when we were interviewing an elderly woman with spasmodic torticollis. The graduate student complimented the woman on how young she looked and how smooth her skin appeared, and the client confessed, "I hate to say it, but both my sister and me have used [the famous hemorrhoidal preparation] for years. It's a miracle worker."

So since the time of Hippocrates, ancient Egypt, and the Ayurvedic healers of ancient India we have grasped and struggled to find remedies for the maladies that defy contemporary treatment. Voltaire was close when he complained that the secrets of remedy are not fully revealed. All we can do is keep learning. And in the meantime try to keep our cat free of hair balls.

REFERENCES

Cures. Retrieved July 30, 2007, from http://www.stat.uga.edu/~molly/remedy.html

Shram, J., & Salmans, S. (2006). *Weird Cures: The most hilarious, disgusting, and downright dangerous medical treatments ever!* Philadelphia: Running Press.

Skeptical Inquirer. Retrieved July 30, 2007, from http://www.csicop.org/

CHAPTER 7

COMPASSION
FATIGUE

Compassion is not religious business, it is human business. It is not luxury, it is essential for our own peace and mental stability. It is essential for human survival.

—Dalai Lama
Head of the Dge-lugs-pa order of Tibetan Buddhists
Nobel Peace Prize, 1989

The dew of compassion is a tear.

—Lord Byron, English poet

Sometimes you have to travel half way around the world to find what's in your own backyard. This past weekend, I was attending a conference of professionals in communication disorders in Napier, a beautiful city on Hawke's Bay on the North Island of New Zealand. The same Hawke's Bay that Captain James Cook named after his hero and mentor Admiral Sir Edward Hawke. In his 1769 journal, Cook noted its majestic mountain backdrop and high white cliffs, but the area soon became another site of violent confrontation between the indigenous Maori and the *pakeha* explorers on Cook's *Endeavour* (Darkin, 2007). Another notable historic and tragic event in this lush current setting of vineyards, art deco buildings, and turquoise water was to take place much later when Napier and surrounds were wracked with a devastating earthquake on February 3, 1931 that took the lives of 256 people. So this setting of great beauty has been the scene of regrettable tragedy as well, once again painting a picture of irony and contrast.

So while enjoying the backdrop of our setting on Hawke's Bay, I made a discovery of my own. Listening to a presentation by Peter Huggard and Sally Kedge (2007) on the topic of burnout in healthcare professionals, I learned about the concepts behind the words *compassion fatigue.* And to my surprise, I found that one of my fellow faculty members at Florida State University, Dr. Charles Figley, has indeed done quite a bit of research and written books on the concept of burnout and compassion fatigue (Figley, 1995, 1997, 2002). Figley has written that the concept of compassion fatigue has been around since 1992 when Joinson used the term in a nursing magazine. It fit the description of a condition reported by nurses working with hospital emergencies. The term *compassion fatigue* indeed seems to be an evolving set of concepts and, although intimately related to the term *burnout,* it is not precisely the same. Figley emphasizes that compassion fatigue is a more user friendly term than what has been proposed by some as secondary traumatic stress disorder, which is nearly identical to posttraumatic stress disorder, except it affects those emotionally affected by the trauma of another (usually a client or a family member). Burnout, countertransference, worker dissatisfaction, and other related concepts are all related to compassion fatigue, and all of these conditions are increasingly becoming recognized as a problem not only for families and caregivers, but also healthcare professionals (Figley, 1995). Compassion fatigue in healthcare providers, especially first responders and emergency medical personnel, and in persons responding to mass disasters (Hurricane Katrina, 9/11, the Southeast Asian tsunami, and the Napier earthquake come to mind) appear affected and at risk. Likewise, healthcare professionals (speech-language pathologists, audiologists, and special education workers come to mind), appear vulnerable to the condition of developing a dilution of compassion as well as a host of related conditions. Substance abuse and the dissolution of personal relationships are too frequently seen in emergency medical personnel and others whose days are filled with working with the suffering. The extent to which those who work with the sufferers suffer is becoming increasingly relevant.

The "cost of caring" is well documented in longterm caregivers of the chronically ill, especially in family members of persons with Alzheimer's disease or other forms of dementia. Likewise, burnout in special education teachers and those working with the profoundly developmentally disabled is widely recognized. How prevalent is this concept in our professions? What can be done to ward it off or avoid it? What work settings or clinical populations appear most related to it? Under what conditions is compassion fatigue most likely to thrive? How is it assessed and treated? These are the questions that Figley, Huggard, and others are wrestling with and hope to clarify. I am fortunate to have stumbled onto these important issues and the inherently imperative concept of compassion fatigue while serving part of my Erskine Fellowship at the University of Canterbury in Christchurch, New Zealand. And behold, one of the world experts on the topic resides at my home base of Florida State University in scenic Tallahassee. I look forward to chatting with and collaborating with Figley, Huggard, and others in order to address the effects of compassion fatigue in our professions.

Lord Byron was right. The dew of compassion may indeed be a tear. But as the Dalai reminds us, it is essential for human survival.

REFERENCES

Darkin, J. (2007). *On Cook's trail: A holiday history of Captain Cook in New Zealand.* Auckland: Reed Publishing Ltd.

Figley, C. R. (Ed.). (1995). *Compassion fatigue: Coping with secondary traumatic stress disorder in those who treat the traumatized.* New York: Brunner/Mazel.

Figley, C. R. (Ed.). (1997). *Burnout in Families: The systemic costs of caring.* New York: CRC Press.

Figley, C. R. (Ed.). (2002). *Treating compassion fatigue.* New York: Brunner-Routledge.

Huggard, P., & Kedge, S. (2007, April). Coping with stress and burnout in a profession: A national survey. Presentation at New Zealand Speech Therapists Association meeting, Napier, NZ.

CHAPTER 8

TINGO

Even if you are on the right track, you'll get run over if you just sit there.

—Will Rogers

Will Rogers and Mark Twain are a couple of the most quotable quibblers that ever graced the stages and pages of the United States. Now, thanks to the mother loads found in the virtual world one can discover massive collections of their wisdom, satire, and unabashed sarcasm. Wrapped in many of those linguistically clever quotes is usually a honey nougat of wisdom. They give you pause; they make you smile; they make you think. Perusal of the archives of both of these clever fellows generates the realization that they both were lovers of words. They loved language in its many forms and were most clever at generating words and images that were a double helix of semantics. They created triple double entendres five times over and no doubt relished doing it. Those who follow these musings in our journal are probably aware that we share that fascination with the twists and coils of words. Especially unusual words; those that make you draw up short and utter an audible "huh!" Perhaps our enthrallment with linguistic agility is born in the roots and daily experiences of our chosen profession; one that has to deal with the stark reality of fractured words and their impact on a person's life.

So we latch onto any fresh treatise on word wonderings, and I am sure that many of our personal libraries are filled with tomes that reveal the nuances and surprises of our mother tongue. Such a book is *The Meaning of Tingo and Other Extraordinary Words from around the World* by Adam Jacot de Boinod (2006). Jacot de Boinod, according to this remarkable book's dustcover, got started on this journey when he peeked into a huge Albanian dictionary and found that there were no fewer than twenty-seven words for types of eyebrow and precisely the same number for varieties of mustache. This original curiosity grew into a passion, if not an obsession, and Jacot de Boinod discovered that there are words out there around the world that describe strange and unbelievable things. He was startled to learn that the Inuit have a need for the word *areodjarekput* which means "to exchange wives for a few days only." We have all encountered, in fact may work with, people who are best described by the Central American Spanish word *ataoso,* "one who seeks problems with everything." No doubt we have served on committees with a *neko-neko,* Indonesian for "one who has a creative idea which only makes things worse." I long needed a word for that. It describes perfectly my attempts to do minor repair work around the house. Invariably in an inspired moment of misperceived competence, I have proclaimed, "I can fix that," and that usually means whatever the object or small appliance is will be broken further or completely trashed during the visit to that do-it-yourself dream world. It started many years ago when my extremely handy Dad would enlist my help on a project only to have to farm me out to accordion practice after I came up with a novel idea that eventually botched the job. A case in point was the two-man operation of the attempt to stretch reach into a barely accessible cubby with my gangly teenage arm sticking a burning tissue up and around the innards of an ancient hot water heater as my Dad turned the petcock to begin the emission of propane gas. The usual course of that drama was about three explosive back flashes that singed my arm before the appliance was relighted. I still have an unrealistic fear of hot water heaters and I swear that during our occasional trips up the folding stairs to our attic as I pass our much safer and up-to-date hot water heater, I hear a faint chuckle. If my Dad knew the word he probably would have said, *neko-neko.*

This little book also fills in the gaps by providing words in foreign tongues for activities and objects that have no common English tag. Siblings have forever generated trouble by practicing *mencolek,* the Indonesian word for touching someone lightly with one finger in order to tease him or her. During aquatic exercise, when our legs get tired we sometimes swim with our hands only, and this is called *honuhonu* in Hawaiian. That's a honu ball game. Along with aquatic activity at the beach, we occasionally engage in *engkonio-mai,* which is ancient Greek for "to sprinkle sand over oneself." The process of writing about these unusual words has made me slightly *přesezený,* Czech for being stiff from sitting in the same position for too long. I guess that can be expected when we start to get *qarba,* the Persian word for white hairs appearing in the beard. Certainly, that is only a male phenomenon though, unless you are a *poti,* a woman with a beard in the Tulu language of India. Back in the 1960s a lot of our friends had *daberlack,* the Northern Ireland name for seaweed or uncontrollable long hair.

A gap in our English dental vocabulary is the space between the teeth. Malaysians have the word *gigi rongak* to refer to it. Displaying the teeth during laughter is called *kashr* in Persian, and a toothsome word that we are unlikely to need is *puccekuli,* the Indian Tulu word for a tooth growing after the eightieth birthday. Another word that we don't have an English equivalent for, but that I've sometimes needed, is *kauhaga moa,* the label of Easter Islanders to designate the first and shortest claw of the chicken. Another one that is hard to work into a conversation is the word *wazahat,* the Persian word for the little bit of sweat and dung attached to a sheep's tail. This is similar to the term *daggies* for *daglocks,* the bits around the tail of a sheep according to Australian and New Zealand street (or rather pasture) slang. In fact, "*Shake your daggies,*" is classic Aussie slang for "get a move on." American Hopi has some interesting words as well, including *musa'ytaka* which is used for insects, airplanes, pilots, and anything that flies with the exception of birds. On many occasion my friend Mick McNeil and I have needed a word such as *kimamu,* the Hawaiian word for fish gathering around a hook that they hesitate to bite.

Foods and eating experiences also generate many words in foreign languages that English does not specify. One restaurant behavior that we rarely see in three-star palaces of cuisine is *slappare,* the evocative Italian word for eating everything, even to the point of licking the plate. The Dutch have a marvelous word, *uitbuiken,* for the process of taking your time at dinner and relaxing. Family dining usually results in an occasional appearance of *sunasor-pok,* the practice of eating what remains of others' food. A Persian word that has a false friend flavor in that it is very close to English slang is *shitta,* the Persian word for food left at night and eaten in the morning. Perhaps that is why that leftover slice of cold pizza consumed for breakfast always tastes like *shitta.* Finally, the Cook Islands Maori have a remarkable reduplicative word, '*akapu'aki'aki*, which signifies the end of a satisfying repast and means to belch repeatedly.

Oh, and *tingo* is a word not likely to be used more than once since it is the Pascuense word from Easter Island that means, "to take all of the objects that one desires from the house of a friend, one at a time, by borrowing them." Some friend. As Mark Twain said, *lingua* planted ever so slightly *en bucca*, "go to heaven for the climate, hell for the company."

I'm sure Mr. Twain would have loved the word *tingo* and relished Jacot de Boinod's book. After all, it was the creator of Tom and Huck himself who stated "the difference between the right word and the almost-right word is the difference between the lightning and the lightning-bug."

REFERENCE

Jacot de Boinod, A. J. (2006). *The meaning of Tingo and other extraordinary words from around the world.* New York: Penguin Press.

CHAPTER 9

BROCA'S BRAIN: BROTHER, WHEREFORE ART THOU?

I washed your brain, but I had trouble getting the think stains out.

—Cindy
(character in *The Adventures of Jimmy Neutron: Boy Genius*, 2002)

The Musée de l'Homme (Museum of Man) was created in 1937 by Paul Rivet, for the splendiferous event of the World's Fair in Paris. Amid the lavishness of the Fair exhibits was Pablo Picasso's *Guernica,* commissioned for the Spanish Pavilion and hailed by many as modern art's most dramatic antiwar statement. The Museum of Man is the descendant of the Musée d'Ethnographie du Trocadéro founded in 1918 and occupies most of the Passy wing of the Palais de Chaillot in the 16th arrondissement. In 1937 the world was boiling with social unrest with the continuing tragedies of the Spanish Civil War (the inspiration for Picasso's mural) as well as the architectural posturing of Soviet and Nazi Germany architects and edifices. The mounting social turmoil did not prevent 32 million visitors from enjoying boat races on the Seine, grand boxing championships, horse racing, and a wine harvesting festival (Herbert, 1998). Ice cream, hamburgers, and fairy floss, reincarnated as cotton candy, were already around and popular thanks to the 1904 St. Louis World's Fair, and the visitors on the banks of the Seine marveled at the Trocadero and Chaillot palace as a perfect repository for a museum dedicated to the natural history of humankind.

Carl Sagan, the Harvard and Cornell researcher and professor of astrophysics who became famous for his popularization of astronomy and debunking of junk science, wrote an influential book in 1979 entitled *Broca's Brain: Reflections on the Romance of Science* (Sagan, 1979). I remember reading that collection of essays in the early 1980s and being enthralled by Sagan's intellect and the breadth of his interests. In fact, one comes across the observation by Isaac Asimov on various Internet sites that Sagan was one of only two people he had ever met who were clearly smarter than Asimov himself. The other was computer and artificial intelligence wizard, Marvin Minsky. I also had the impression that Sagan was a profound intellect and was amazed at his appearances on the American late night television show with Johnny Carson by his ability to pique interest in remarkably highbrow and philosophical subject matter. *Broca's Brain* was an immensely popular crossover best seller in the 1980s. It set Sagan up for further writing that earned him a Pulitzer Prize as well as a sojourn to Hollywood to work on the adaptation of his book *Contact* for a film with Jody Foster. Although his manner of speech (particularly his pronunciation of "billions and billions") became fodder for many standup comedians, those in the scientific community never doubted or tarnished Sagan's remarkable contributions.

So it came to pass that Carl Sagan rhapsodized in *Broca's Brain* about the exquisite experience of standing in the Musée de l'Homme as he contemplated and gazed upon the preserved brain of Pierre Paul Broca (June 28, 1824–July 9, 1880) the scientific giant of the 19th century who contributed so much of what we know about the localization of articulate speech in the brain of humans. Broca was a French physician, anthropologist, and eventually a senator who believed that by studying the brains of cadavers and correlating the known experiences and behaviors of the former possessor of the organs, human behavior could be revealed, associated with brain function, and better understood. For that purpose he collected hundreds of human brains in jars of the preservative formalin. Upon his death in 1880 with exquisite irony, his own brain was preserved in formalin and added to the collection in the museum, along with hundreds of skulls that Broca had used in his comparative cephalametric studies. When Sagan happened upon Broca's brain in the museum, along with Broca's milestone patient "Tan" Leborgne, he was awestruck by the irony of it all. Here was Broca, for whom the region of the frontal lobe of the cortex that he had described was subsequently named, with his own Broca's area discernible. Sagan was mesmerized by the incongruity of all of this. In *Broca's Brain* he used that visit to the Museum of Man to launch philosophical questions that challenge some core ideas of human existence and consciousness such as *How much of that man known as Paul Broca can still be found in this jar?*

Because of this recollection of Sagan's fascination with Broca's and Leborgne's brains and consistent with a professional mild case of celebrity worship (so I have a personalized license plate that says *Broca*; doesn't everyone?), I was eager on a recent professional visit to Paris to visit the Musée de l'Homme and reflect as Sagan did, upon Broca's area in Broca's very brain. It was not to be. Brother Broca, wherefore art thou?

As it happened, I was visiting Paris with two friends and colleagues, Dr. Mike Theodoros, a renowned Australian psychiatrist, and his wife Dr. Deborah Theodoros, a renowned Australian speech-language pathologist at the University of Queensland. My wife Corinne, a renowned wife and gerontology health-care professional accompanied us. All were keen to join me on my visit to the shadows of the Eiffel Tower to search for the brain of Broca in the Museum of Man. Our first visit had to be aborted. The museum was closed (Monday closing), but an employee graciously informed us that "all neurologique material including brains has been transferred to the newly opened Quai Branly museum." We were informed, "cross the river, turn left at the Eiffel Tower, go a couple of blocks, you can't miss it."

We set out again, and after a walk along the Seine enjoyed the modern architecture of the recently opened Branly museum, along with its most unique "living wall" (200m long by 12m tall) on part of the exterior of the museum. This botanic wall was designed and planted by Patrick Blanc. Seeing the exotic plants and vines covering the walls of the new museum was as unique as the exhibits of indigenous art, cultures, and civilizations from Africa, Asia, Oceania, and the Americas. With barely contained enthusiasm we purchased tickets and inquired at the information desk as to where we would find the neurological exhibits and Broca's brain in particular. We were met with a response that clearly indicated that we might as well have asked to see the corpse of Edith Piaf. After more inquiry and the assurance by a museum administrator that there were absolutely no exhibits or holdings on topics European, we were informed that no registration of "Broca" was currently encrypted on the Branly master computer list. A kindly employee suggested that we had been misinformed and that Broca certainly was still housed at the Museum of Man.

The hour was late and the brasseries were calling, so we redirected our efforts and vowed to continue the next day on this now rather mystifying search for the missing Broca's brain. Upon our revisit to the Musée de l'Homme, we went directly to an information desk and explained that we were in search of Broca's brain and had been misdirected to the new Branly museum whose administrators insisted that the collection had not been moved and indeed resided in its original home. After referral to two levels of supervisory inquiry we were met with very helpful staff who invited us to their private coffee-break room behind the scenes and informed us that they would attempt to contact one of the principal curators at the museum, who currently was on his day off work. They indeed contacted the curator who in fact promised to come in on his day off and help us search for Broca's brain. In less than 30 minutes, Dr. Philippe Mennecier, a linguist and researcher on Inuit dialects and languages of Greenland was at our service and kindly asked how he could help. He informed us that they indeed had an extensive collection of Broca's work, in fact 83 cabinets of skulls, death masks, and cephalametric artifacts, but he was unaware of the museum's holding of either Broca's or Leborgne's brain. He kindly took us to his most unique office however, and offered to search his data bases more thoroughly. As he searched, he invited us to step outside his office through an office window that led to a remarkable arched terrace with an absolutely astonishing view of the Eiffel Tower. After a bit, he invited us back into his office and said that in all likelihood the brains of Broca and Leborgne were now in the Dupuytren Museum at the College of Medicine of the University of Paris.

Dr. Philippe Mennecier proceeded then to invite us to a behind-the-scenes tour of the collections of Broca as well as those of Franz Josef Gall, the infamous neurologist and phrenologist who advocated that character of people could be discerned by reading their cranial configuration and bumps on the head. We spent a fascinating 2 hours in the company of Dr. Mennecier as he opened cabinet after cabinet to display the skull casts and death masks of hundreds of individuals who had been measured and studied by Broca or by Gall. Casts of criminals, famous composers (Franz Liszt et al.), intellectuals, and an assortment of saints and sinners were revealed as Dr. Mennecier unlocked the cabinets of cranial history. Our guide was most helpful and gracious and we are indebted to him for a remarkable journey into the 19th century and the starch-colored world of Broca and Gall. We did not find the preserved brains of Broca or Leborgne this time, but further detective work has all but convinced us that on the next trip to Paris we will head straight to the Dupuytren Museum and gaze upon the wonders that so fascinated Carl Sagan as he contemplated Broca's brain and all of its ramifications to neuroscience and that greatest gift of all, human language.

REFERENCES

Amunts, K. (2006). *Broca's region.* International Brain Research Organization. Retrieved from Internet on October 29, 2006 from http://www.ibro.org/Pub_Main_Display.asp?Main_ID=15

Broca, P. (1861a). Perte de la parole, ramollissement chronique et desstruction partielle du lob antérieur gauche de cerveau. *Bulletins de la Société d'Anthropologie, 62,* 235–238.

Broca, P. (1861b). Remarques sur le siége de la faculté du langage articulé, suiv-ies d'une observation d'aphe-mie (Perte de la Parole). *Bulletins et memoires de la Societe Anatomique de Paris, 36,* 330–357.

Broca, P. (1863). Localisation des fonctions cérébrales. Siege du langage articulé. *Bulletins de la Société d'Anthropologie Séance du 2 Auril, 1863, 200*–204.

Broca, P (1865). Sur la siege de la faculté langage articulé. *Bulletin of the Society of Anthropology, 6,* 377–396.

Herbert, J. D. (1998). *Paris 1937: Worlds on exhibition.* Ithaca, NY: Cornell University.

Sagan, C. (1979). *Broca's brain: Reflections on the romance of science.* New York: Random House.

CHAPTER 10

COOK AND KIWI

He aha te mea nui? What is the greatest thing? *He tangata!*
It is people. *He tangata!*

—Maori Aphorism

On June 30, 1768 Lt. James Cook received his orders from the British Royal Society and the Royal Navy to begin the first of his three incredible voyages to the South Pacific. He and his crew of 94 were to launch an expedition of exploration, cartography, and scientific research. It was the Age of Enlightenment in Europe, and science and exploration were revered values. The soon-to-be Captain James Cook received three pages of handwritten orders, including a charge to observe and record in Tahiti an astrological event, the Transit of Venus. But there was more. Apart from the standard British Admiralty crew for a sailing ship—officers, midshipmen, and craftsmen—also on board was a group of civilians led by an aristocratic and wealthy 25-year-old naturalist, Joseph Banks. With the fervor of the Enlightenment motivating them, Banks and his team of scientists, artists, and servants collected and began recording aspects of plant and animal life from the exotic realms that had never before been seen in Europe. Later, after their travels and mapping of the east coast of Australia, imagine the consternation and incredulity generated by descriptions and drawings of the kangaroo and platypus. Some thought the platypus was a hoax. The scientists also were charged with conducting anthropological investigation of the peoples and cultures they encountered. A major accomplishment, after the Transit of Venus was duly recorded in Tahiti, was the tribulation of exploring the east coast of Australia. Prior to leaving on the quest for terra australis incognita, the Endeavour circumnavigated the islands of New Zealand and though Cook made a cartographic error by showing the Banks Peninsula as an island, he constructed an astonishingly detailed and accurate map of New Zealand (Captain Cook Society, 2006).

The comparison of Cook's rendering with a present-day satellite photograph can be appreciated in juxtaposition on a beautifully mounted presentation at Paul Arnold's Antique Print Gallery on New Regent Street in Christchurch (www.antiquemaps.co.nz). We spent a pleasant afternoon perusing old maps and drawings of the Cook era with the proprietor and engaged in fascinating conversation about various interpretations of Captain Cook's death at Kealakekua Bay in the Sandwich Islands, which were later to be called Hawaii. Mr. Arnold alerted me to the new version of Cook's voyage by Dame Anne Salmond of the University of Auckland.

After Captain Cook's remarkable discoveries and mapmaking of Australia and New Zealand he returned to Britain and was hailed as a hero and celebrity. Subsequently, he undertook two other significant voyages of discovery. On the second voyage he explored and circumnavigated Antarctica and described the amazing "ice mountains" floating in the frigid waters. His third and final voyage from 1776–1780 was marked by the exploration and mapping of the Sandwich Islands (Hawaii) and remarkably, even a part of the coast of North America while searching for a northern passage between the Pacific and Atlantic Oceans.

After his tragic and controversial death at Kealakekua Bay, precipitated by his tactless retaliation for the theft of one of his long boats, it is alleged that parts of his body were boiled, distributed, and eaten by the offended residents of the islands. Some of the intact fragments of his body, including his uniquely scarred right hand, were returned by the islanders and buried at sea, and his crew completed their journey back to England.

The voyages of Captain Cook are preserved in many historical accounts and make for fascinating reading. It is even possible to access the actual ship logs of Captain Cook and Joseph Banks and relive their daily adventures and impressions. The *Endeavour Journal* can be accessed from several sources on the Internet, including a national library repository in Australia that displays photographs of the actual pages of the handwritten journals of Captain Cook, Joseph Banks, and the ship's surgeon (Australian National Library, 2006).

A recent comprehensive exploration of this unique historical era is contained in a sensitive and unbiased treatment of the cultural effects of the encounters between Cook and the indigenous peoples of the South Seas. The tome is written by an eminent scholar from the University of Auckland by the name of Dame Anne Salmond. The intriguing title of the book is *The Trial of the Cannibal Dog: The Remarkable Story of Captain Cook's Encounters in the South Seas* (Salmond, 2003). This work supersedes and provides much more of a nonjudgmental anthropological perspective on the clash of cultures and peoples than do previous books about Cook, including a capstone work by a scholar with the evocative name of J. C. Beaglehole (1992).

The magnificent islands of New Zealand were some of the last pieces of land to be settled. Of course, the Maori indigenous people were there before Captain Cook and his crew recorded their sometimes feisty, sometimes cordial encounters with this group of inhabitants of *Aotearoa*, the Land of the Long White Cloud. Archaeological and linguistic evidence (Sutton, 1994) suggests that probably several waves of migration occurred from Eastern Polynesia to New Zealand between 800 and 1300 AD. The first voyage of Cook and company was to reflect the interactions of Europeans and indigenous peoples throughout history. Along with trinkets, new diseases were passed on to the "natives," and exploitation and cultural dilution were activated. Beads, iron nails, and tuberculosis were dispensed with alacrity. The Maori population declined precipitously, and against the backdrop of bloody intertribal warfare, musket wars, and the insinuation of the values and religions of missionaries, the Maori culture was deeply jeopardized. Fortunately, stabilization evolved and today, despite persistent social and economic ills, a cultural revival exists. The language, crafts, and art of the Maori is evident nearly everywhere in the Land of the Long White Cloud.

The remarkable hospitality and affability of the inhabitants of New Zealand was evident to my sister Marybeth, my wife Corinne, and me on a recent invited visit to the South Island. The New Zealand Speech-Language Therapists' Association held their biennial conference in Christchurch, and I was privileged to present a couple of lectures to the group. The opening ceremony was drenched in the respect and culture of the Maori people of New Zealand. We participated with grateful enjoyment in a traditional welcome practiced by the Maori. This welcome or *powwhiri* includes oratory, songs, and a welcoming *hongi*. This is the traditional greeting that includes the gentle pressing together of the nose and forehead. The *hongi* represents welcome and acceptance. Often this is performed three times: the first pressing is a greeting to the person, the second acknowledges ancestors, and a third pressing of nose and forehead honors life in this world. In the *hongi*, the *ha* or breath of life is exchanged and intermingled. Through the exchange of this physical greeting, one is no longer considered *manuhiri* (visitor) but rather *tangata whenua*, one of the people of the land for the duration of the visit.

We felt enriched and welcome indeed. New Zealand is a land of magnificent beauty and a rich diversity of cultures. The Maori presence and influence saturates the society. This country is a land of societal values many of us could take a lesson from (genuine respect for and protection of the environment, a highly prioritized national focus on human welfare and benevolence, and less obsession with competition and the compulsive pursuit of coinage). But the soul of the Land of the Long White Cloud is the people. What is the greatest thing? *He tangata.* It is people. *He tangata!*

REFERENCES

Australian National Library. Retrieved May 2, 2006 from http://www.nla.gov.au/apps/cdview?pi=nla.msmsl-t-cd

Beaglehole, J. C. et al. (1992). *The life of Captain James Cook*. Palo Alto: Stanford University Press.

Captain Cook Society. Retrieved May 2, 2006 from http://www.CaptainCookSociety.com

Salmond, A. (2003). *The trial of the cannibal dog: The remarkable story of Captain Cook's encounters in the South Seas*. New Haven and London: Yale University Press.

Sutton, Douglas G. (Ed.). (1994). *The origins of the first New Zealanders*. Auckland: Auckland University Press.

CHAPTER 11

CELL HELL

The cell phone has transformed public places into giant phone-a-thons in which callers exist within narcissistic cocoons of private conversations.

—Mary Schmich

1983 was a memorable year. In the United States, Alice Walker won the Pulitzer Prize for fiction for *The Color Purple*. Film goers reveled in the story and sound track of the movie, "The Big Chill," and, in an omen of things to come, Michael Jackson hit it big with "Beat It." Tragically, a Korean Airlines passenger airliner was shot down for straying into Soviet airspace. Another event in the "things don't change much" category was the U.S. invasion of the island of Granada.

Big things were happening in the world of technology as well. In 1983, Motorola introduced DynaTAC, the first truly mobile telephone, and by the end of that year, the first commercial cellular phone systems were being used in Chicago and in the Baltimore/Washington, D.C. area. The world has rarely witnessed such an avalanche of technological advancement for the masses over the span of the following years. In a thoughtful article in *The New Atlantis: A Journal of Technology and Society* entitled "Our Cell Phones, Ourselves" Christine Rosen (2004) has penned a provocative historical tracing and social commentary on the impact of cell phone use on society. Some of her carefully researched musings are unnerving. It is hard to come away from the article without growing concern that we may be experiencing a significant change in the effects of technology on societal customs and traditions.

We hear daily of the vocal rumblings of discontent with the discourtesy and downright boorishness of public cell phone users. With the increase and near saturation of cell phone use (according to Rosen [2004] there are a billion cell phone users worldwide, and sometime between 2010 and 2020 anyone who can afford a cell phone will have one), we are witnessing a transformation of society and of social interaction in public places.

The horror stories abound. Cell phone disruptions on trains, planes, doctor's offices, grocery stores, book stores, libraries, church and synagogue services, and even funerals and weddings. Nearly everyone reports being annoyed by poor cell phone etiquette, and offenders are everywhere. We are Jeckyle and Hydes when it comes to being the annoyed or the annoyer. In the immortal words of the comic strip possum, Pogo, "We have met the enemy, and they are us."

Concerts, plays, and films are interrupted by cell rings; one report related an incident of a cell phone ringing that seemed to come from the casket of the recently embalmed. It turns out it was the misplaced phone, of a funeral parlor employee, that had slipped onto the satin next to the guest of honor. The only thing that surpasses the annoyance of a cell phone disruption during a public event is to have to endure the inane varieties of ring tones that are available. Selecting a revving Harley-Davidson, Meow-Mix TV jingle, or some misogynistic, barely intelligible rap "lyric" are all reasons for doing extra time in the deeper recesses of hell. Tartarus, that special waiting room in Hell reserved for the punishment of worst offenders, is too good for anyone with a ring tone of "Achy Breaky Heart."

Lest readers think this is the ranting of an unmitigated curmudgeon, it must be pointed out that cell phone annoyance is nearly universal. The *Zagat* restaurant guide reports that cell phone rudeness is the number one complaint of diners. Rosen (2004) also reports a survey that indicates that 59% of respondents would rather visit the dentist than sit next to someone using a cell phone.

What are the topics of these ever so necessary phone conversations? Are they truly emergencies, parenting necessities, or other safety concerns? Mostly not. The majority of conversations seem to revolve around seemingly unnecessary progress reports. "Guess where I am?" "I'm in the car, Honey; I'm only about two blocks from home now. I just passed Home Depot." "I'm in the produce section. Right by the broccoli. Oh, did I tell you I had another of my little 'accidents' today? Do we still have some Immodium left or should I pick up some more."

If truth were known, it appears that the motivation for much cell phone talk is what some have referred to as "peacocking." Strutting around with feathers and the latest technology displayed loudly and prominently to communicate to all around them, either "Look what I have. Am I not indispensable and ever so important?" Or, "Don't you think I would be a wonderful mate? If you are attracted to me, you can be sure that you would pass on the absolute finest quality gene pool as evidenced by my Blackberry or video-camera-text messaging-iPod downloading-salad shooter state-of-the-art phone." As Rosen (2004) puts it, "Men are using their mobile phones as peacocks use their immobilizing feathers and male bullfrogs use their immoderate croaks: To advertise to females their worth, status, and desirability."

Some national and regional differences appear to exist regarding cell phone abuse and pollution. Israel residents are reported to use the cell phone four times more than Americans, and there is a 76% saturation rate of the population of Israel who are mobile phone users. Two Israeli sociologists reported there were no fewer than 10 cell phone interruptions during a recent staging of *One Flew Over the Cuckoo's Nest* at Israel's National Theater. Their report was subtitled "Chutzpah and chatter in the Holy Land." In Taiwan, nearly everyone who has ears and hands has a mobile phone, and there is a fear by some that a process of evolutionary fusing of phone to pinna will emerge in future generations. Rosen (2004) reports that studies of regional differences in the United States show that cell phone users in the South are "more likely to turn their phones off in church." However, a cleric in our town is reported to have announced recently, "No text messaging during church services." Users in the Western states are most likely to turn their cell phones off in theaters, libraries, concerts, and schools.

Is this technologically induced change in societal behavior merely an annoyance or a harbinger of the erosion of the rules of social interaction and communication? The research on the topic is not all negative. One cross-cultural study of Taiwanese and American university students found that heavy users of mobile phones in both cultures reported significantly better personal relationships with friends and family as well as higher academic achievement (Chen & Lever, 2005).

Much of the news is not positive, though. An increasing number of studies report concern over the social consequences of heavy, even addictive, cell phone use. Sociologists are beginning to express distress about degradation of face-to-face communication in the presence of virtual communication. According to Rosen (2004), Kenneth J. Gergen has argued that one reason cell phones allow a peculiar form of diversion in public spaces is that they encourage "absent presence," a state where "one is physically present but is absorbed by a technologically mediated world of elsewhere."

We witness examples of *absent presence* everywhere and every day. My early concerns about the hazards of cell phone use during driving (one of our studies found a 28% decrease across several parameters of reaction time and cognition while talking on a cell phone) are being joined by the *absent presence* of pedestrians who amble along chatting. Every day we see near misses on our campus. Students step off the curb while jabbering nearly into the path of drivers. Attentional resource allocation has its limits, as many of us know, and when most of the attentional pool is diverted to finding out "Wassup?" little remains for shared tasks, such as walking safely.

An increasing occurrence of social isolation and general bad manners is the practice of people in line at the grocery store or the post office who are so deep into their own conversations that they do not offer even the most basic pleasantries or courtesy to the salesperson or cashier. Wherever we find the co-incidental gatherings of strangers, it is now most common to witness immersion into the sea of me and cell phone and little effort to relate face-to-face to real, present humans. Many people who study these things are concerned that we are trading virtual connection for face-to-face social isolation. This difficulty harmonizing virtual and real social engagement is altering social etiquette. We can expect more incidents of people being escorted off airplanes, kicked out of movie theaters, and exiled from lectures and concerts due to the blossoming rudeness and obliviousness that seems to be accompanying the increase in cell phone use.

What is to come of all this? Just as social mores have changed relative to spitting in public spittoons and cigarette smoking in confined public spaces, perhaps society will evolve to incorporate sensible solutions to the growing annoyances of cell phone barbarianism. As Rosen (2004) has so aptly put it, cell phones provide us with a new, but not necessarily superior means of communicating with each other. They encourage talk, but we're losing the gentle art of public social conversation. These necessary little instruments of the devil link us to those we know, but remove us from the strangers who surround us in public space. Our constant accessibility and frequent exchange of information is certainly useful and most important in times of emergency. But the overwhelming majority of its use is limited to ultra-superficial variations on the theme of *Was-sup?* and *Where are you?* It surely would be a terrible irony if "being connected" encouraged and resulted in a disconnection from community life. We need no further erosion of the spontaneous encounters and everyday decencies that make society both civilized and tolerable.

Can you hear me now?

REFERENCES

Chen, & Lever, K. (2005). *Relationships among mobile phones, social networks, and academic achievement: A comparison of US and Taiwanese college students*. Report: School of Communication, Information, and Library Studies, New Brunswick University, accessed January 31, 2006, from http://mobile.ris .org/main/baza/baza.php?bid=397

Rosen, C. (2004). Our cell phones, ourselves. *The New Atlantis, 6,* 26–45.

CHAPTER 12

PROFANITY

*Under certain circumstances, profanity provides a relief denied
even to prayer.*

—Mark Twain

Oh heck! Another doggone pet mess. As our local revered football coach might say, "Dadgum it! Seems like it's just one dadgum thing after another." Makes you want to curse, cuss, swear, blaspheme, or utter an obscenity.

Profanity has been around probably as long as language and serves a variety of interesting social, emotional, and linguistic functions. Psycholinguistic studies have demonstrated that profanity and other obscene words produce physical effects in people who read or hear them, such as an elevated cardiac rate, increased Galvanic skin response, blushing, trembling, shallow breathing, and in extreme cases loss of normally regulated bowel and bladder function. Some words are so intertwined with emotional connotation that they just make you want to sh . . . well, you get the idea. This essay will not be a parade of all of the well known taboo words, as cathartic as that might be, but rather will attempt to explore some of the nuances of taboo words across time and cultures.

Swearing has not eluded scholars as a topic of titillating research. Researchers have explored ingeniously the perception and processing of swear words. In one study, scientists started with the frequently used Stroop test, during which subjects are flashed a series of words written in different colors and are asked to react by calling out the colors of the words rather than the words themselves. We use variants of this test in our laboratory to study cognitive processing time and inhibition of attention. In the Stroop, if participants see the word "chair" written in yellow letters, they are supposed to say "yellow." In the study of Stroop reaction time and profanity, researchers inserted a number of obscenities and vulgarities in the standard word list. Charting participants' immediate and delayed responses, researchers found that, first of all, people needed significantly more time to call out the colors of the curse words than they did for neutral terms like chair. The experience of seeing emotion-tinged words apparently distracted the participants from the color-coding task at hand.

Emotions and words are interrelated and although sociocultural modifications in the emotional responses to obscenity evolves, we can readily identify a corpus of words that cannot, as George Carlin so aptly put it years ago, be said on TV. These nonbroadcast words have been affectionately dubbed, "S, P, F, C, C, M, and T." Carlin's rants on language and taboo words worked its way through the court system until in 1978 the Supreme Court of the United States upheld the right of broadcasters to censor the list from broadcast during times of the day when there was a reasonable risk that children might be in the audience. Before Carlin, Lenny Bruce, an American comedian, had been arrested and taken to court for using some of the same words in his standup comedy routine. Carlin has since expanded this list by three or four words, but broadcast standards have changed to the point where a few of these "list" words are now regularly heard on mainstream broadcasts and all of them, plus some 14-carat hybrids, are heard on U.S. cable television.

What is it about profanity that has maintained it as so endearing and persistent, if not completely civilized? Cursing and profanity seems to be a human universal. Every language or dialect ever analyzed by linguists, be the language living or dead or spoken by hoards or by a small tribe in the Amazon basin, seems to have a lexicon that is well seasoned with forbidden words, many of which are some variant on comedian Carlin's famous list of the seven dirty words.

Geoffrey Hughes (1993) has written an academic and properly researched tome on this seemingly fascinating topic. His book *Swearing: A Social History of Foul Language, Oaths and Profanity in English* is a good starting point for scholars who want to dig into the history and evolution of nasty words. A rich archive of other works, some scholarly, some designed for street consumption, is readily available from Amazon.com and other purveyors of printed prurience. How about this for a list of references for your term paper:

English as a Second F*cking Language: How to Swear Effectively, Explained in Detail with Numerous Examples Taken From Everyday Life by Sterling Johnson (1996), New York: St. Martins Press.

Depraved and Insulting English by Peter Novobatzky (2002, New York: Harvest Books).

Watch Your F*cking Language: How to Swear Effectively, Explained in Explicit Detail and Enhanced by Numerous Examples Taken From Everyday Life by Sterling Johnson (2004).

The Anatomy of Swearing by Ashley Montague (2001), Philadelphia University of Pennsylvania Press.

Cursing in America: A Psycholinguistic Study of Dirty Language in the Courts, in the Movies, in the Schoolyards and on the Streets by Timothy Jay (1992), Philadelphia: John Benjamin.

Profanity can be interesting when crosslinguistic obscenity use is considered. Many commonalities exist across languages. Some authors have speculated that while swearing in German and several other languages seems to focus predominantly on elimination and variants of poop, in English most swearing appears to be sexual in nature. Blasphemy and sacrilege appear to be waning, though it was prominent in the writing of Shakespeare ("Zounds!" a contraction of "God's wounds;" and "Gadzooks!" a derivation of "God's hooks," or crucifixion).

Of course, social context is a great determinant of the amount of profanity that is used. In certain informal social situations, swearing is used as sort of a symbolic communication of bonding. Although some retain the idea that swearing is conducted mostly by coarse, crude, or lower-class individuals, ample evidence exists that swearing knows no rigid class structure. Kings, heads of state (Lyndon Baynes Johnson was notorious for his salty language), and even the clergy have been known to use swear words liberally. One obscure Internet source even catalogs swear words hypothetically used by Jesus Christ (e.g., "Me!" "Me, Mom, and Mom's husband!").

We are all familiar with certain euphemisms used to swear in polite company: "Heck" and "darn" have an old-fashioned ring to them, but people have seemingly always flirted with the boundaries of profanity just as our dadgummed football coach does. "Gosh Almighty," "Gee," "Jiminy Cricket," and "Jumping Jehosephat" are all rather archaic, quaint linguistic ways of not stepping in it. One of the revered elders of my home town of Channing, Waldemar Hanson, occasionally and not without great provocation would cut loose with "By the Great Horn Spoon." To this day I scratch my head at that one and its possible derivation. My Dad used to tell a story about one of his colorful teenage friends whose language was so salty that "he could swear in fractions." On questioning, my Dad would delight in giving an example. ("He'd say 'c***s***er and a half'.")

Some euphemisms have become so commonplace that most people don't even consider them euphemisms. "Little boys' room" is a little over the top for most, but many of us retain use of the euphemistic "bathroom" or "restroom" or "washroom" with no primary objective of bathing, resting, or washing. Most people intend to use a bathroom to "whiz," or "drop the kids off at the pool." Even the term "toilet" is a euphemism, though one notices a reluctance to use the term "toilet" on signs in the United States as opposed to liberal use of this signage in the United Kingdom or Australia. "Toilet" is derived from a French word meaning a shaving cloth and evolved to refer to a washing-up room and finally to its current meaning.

I'm sure Mark Twain would agree that after hitting your thumb with a hammer euphemisms do not provide nearly as much relief as a good, old fashioned, gold-plated polysyllabic swear word. Maybe even with a fraction added. Profanity remains an intriguing aspect of sociolinguistics, and its frequent retention even in people who have neurological damage and an impoverished lexicon remains fertile ground for research. The copralalia of Tourette's syndrome and the evocations of those who are profoundly aphasic reflect this need to understand profanity at more than a blushing level (Brown & Kushner, 2001).

Rude? Inappropriate? Degrading? Uncouth? It depends on the social context and the cochlea of the beholder. Damn right.

REFERENCES

Brown, K. E., & Kushner, H. I. (2001). Eruptive voices: Coprolalia, malediction, and the poetics of cursing. *New Literary History*, 32(3), 573–562.

Hughes, G. (1993). *Swearing: A social history of foul language, oaths and profanity in English*. City, State: Publisher's name.

Jay, T. (2002). *Cursing in America: A psycholinguistic study of dirty language in the courts, in the movies, in the schoolyards and on the streets*. Philadelphia: John Benjamins Publishing Co.

Johnson, S. (1996). *English as a second f*cking language: How to swear effectively, explained in detail with numerous examples taken from everyday life*. New York: St. Martin's Press.

Johnson, S. (2004). *Watch your f*cking language: how to swear effectively, explained in explicit detail and enhanced by numerous examples taken from everyday Life*. New York: St. Martin's Press.

Montague, A. (2001). *The anatomy of swearing*. Philadelphia: University of Pennsylvania Press.

Novobatzky, P. (2002). *Depraved and insulting English*. New York: Harvest Books.

CHAPTER 13

X-RAY EYES

I cannot give any scientist of any age better advice than this: **the intensity of a conviction that a hypothesis is true has no bearing on whether it is true.** *The importance of the strength of our conviction is only to provide a proportionately strong incentive to find out if the hypothesis will stand up to critical examination.*

—Peter B. Medawar, zoologist and immunologist
Advice to a Young Scientist, 1979

X-ray eyes have been an intriguing concept for a long time. I remember well the ads in the comic books of a cartoon man with carefully drawn large glasses that allowed him to see through his hand to reveal bones and internal structures. How intriguing. Many of us who followed our superheroes and perused these ads were on the edge of inference. The unstated possibility was that perhaps these magic glasses would not only allow an educational observation of the magnificent structures of the human body, but might also, through some optic refractory quirk, allow a vision of intact body parts beneath the poodle skirts and Peter Pan blouses of our classmates. I will not admit to having purchased such a magical device as X-ray glasses, but I will say that most of the cheap junk ordered from comic book ads proved to be items for the burying ground of unfulfilled promises and tawdry misrepresentation. They didn't work. The X-ray glasses were a hoax. Revelation of the bio-mysteries would be deferred to another day.

In fact, as pointed out by Skolnick (2005) in an issue of *Skeptical Inquirer*, it was only a little more than a century ago that the German physicist Wilhelm Roentgen startled the world with his discovery of an invisible form of radiation that could result in photographs of the bones and organs beneath the flesh of a living body.

It was November 8, 1895 when Roentgen worked in his darkened Wurzburg laboratory and stumbled onto something that would revolutionize medicine. Roentgen experimented on light phenomena and other emissions generated by discharging electrical currents in glass tubes. His fiddling with cathode rays in glass tubes led him to experiment with assessing the range of the rays beyond the confines of the tubes. To what must have been his astonishment, he noted that when his cardboard-shrouded tube was charged, an object on the other side of the room began to glow. Historians know little about the sequence of Roentgen's work over the next few days, except for his reports that while holding materials between the tube and a screen to test the new rays, he saw the bones of his hand clearly displayed against an outline of flesh. Imagine the wonder and disbelief that this German physicist must have experienced. He immersed himself in isolated work frenzy in his laboratory and refined his observations into reports and scholarly publications. His first reports of these mysterious "X rays" were looked upon askance and even regarded as a hoax by some of his contemporaries, but just 6 years after his remarkable laboratory luck and work, he was awarded the first Nobel Prize in physics in 1901.

Then along came Natasha Demkina, the girl with the X-ray eyes. This teenager from Saransk, Russia, claims to possess X-ray vision that allows her to see inside human bodies. She has been using this vision to make remarkable medical diagnoses that are claimed to be more accurate than those of traditional medical practitioners. As the online periodical Pravda (Jan. 14, 2004) states, she has a gift of "dual vision" that allows her to see and interpret internal body parts without external X ray or ultrasound. According to the Pravda article, Natasha is capable of distinguishing even the tiniest pathology on a molecular level in the deepest corners of a human body, which are usually left undetected by regular ultrasound. "It's like having double vision. I can switch from one to the other in no time if I need to know a person's health problem. I see an entire human organism. It is difficult to explain how I determine specific illnesses. There are certain impulses that I feel from the damaged organs. The secondary vision works only in daytime and is asleep at night."

Claims of empirical testing of Natasha's X-ray eyes have resulted in mostly anecdotal evidence and the testimonials by a growing number of patients, doctors, journalists, and others who have witnessed her diagnoses. According to Skolnick, her increasing following is proving lucrative. The young psychic seems to have an active practice. She reportedly charges the equivalent of approximately $13 per reading and can do about 10 readings each weekday. This provides an income of about $2,600 per month and is more than 40 times the average monthly income of government workers in her home town (Skolnick, 2005).

The May/June edition of *Skeptical Inquirer* has an intriguing set of articles on "Testing Natasha," "Natasha Demkina: The Girl with the Normal Eyes," and "Psychic Swindlers." After designing a protocol and generating a number of carefully controlled experiments on the Girl with the X-Ray Eyes, it was concluded that Natasha's performance did not meet the tester's criteria for success. It was concluded that Natasha may well have developed those skills of other alleged "psychics" that allow clues and careful observation to be molded into generalities about possible "medical conditions." Apparently, the Discovery Channel has produced a program that may be broadcast in the United States that extracts several of Natasha's accurate guesses about undetected medical conditions. No doubt the screening of that show and other programs that continue to dumb down science and follow the sensational trail of alien autopsies, psychokinetic powers, and other claims of the paranormal will attract nonskeptical believers. Pseudoscience is rampant and continues to captivate not only the general public but even politicians and policy makers. P.T. Barnum was probably right, "There's a sucker born every minute."

Despite unprecedented advances in technology and telecommunication, we are a general society, our skeptics tell us, that demonstrates an ongoing love affair with pseudoscience. Scientific literacy seems to be waging an uphill battle against the spewing of sensationalism, reductionism, and bad science that fills our airwaves and sells tabloids. Flim-flaw "X-ray glasses" and the magical powers of teenagers with "X-ray eyes" need to be exposed for the fraudulent hoaxes and superstition they are. Roentgen would be proud.

REFERENCES

Medawar, P. (1979). *Advice to a young scientist.* New York: Harper & Row.

Pravda RU. (2005). Girl with the x-ray eyes. Retrieved July 25, 2005, http://english.pravda.ru/science/19/ 94/377/11797_phenomenon.html

Skolnick, A. (2005). Natasha Demkina: The girl with the normal eyes. *Skeptical Inquirer, 29*(3), 34–37.

CHAPTER 14

MIXED METAPHORS

Take time to stop and smell the tunnel at the end of the rainbow.

—Gary Swing (2005)

anguage is wonderful when it facilitates communication. Language is maddening or hilarious when it fails to do so or gets in the way. Language mavens, as so many of us fancy ourselves, retain and frequently revisit personal collections of fractured language examples for our amusement. Many of these examples are saved from the utterances heard as we go about our daily interactions with people. A rich mother lode is provided by those who endure occasional linguistic scrambling because of stroke, dementia, or traumatic brain injury. "Your very *begoing* today, Nancy," said one of our beloved patients, meaning to compliment a clinician on her very *becoming* new hairstyle. Or a former mortician who became aphasic attempted to explain a proverb by saying, "Don't put all your eggs in one casket."

Difficulty with nonliteral interpretations and use of language has been implicated for a number of years with functions associated with the right cerebral hemisphere. Our colleagues Hiram Brownell and Penny Myers as well as many others have written extensively about the role of the right hemisphere in the use and wreckage of metaphor. Blake (2005) described many of the challenges with figurative or nonliteral language faced by people who have experienced right hemisphere damage. Other writers have associated nonliteral language anomaly with other clinical populations such as people with schizophrenia or "social-pragmatic" disorders (Botting, 1998; Frow, 2001).

Metaphor is a marvelous device that facilitates understanding of complex issues and creates evocative responses to the printed or spoken word. This language tool can be used to balance and enhance discrete linguistic concepts. A carefully crafted metaphor consists of verbal images connecting one impression to something it cannot be. It allows us to substitute one kind of notion with another, usually one that is more familiar. Metaphor use is a form of mental cartography that makes complex ideas easier to navigate. As our late colleague Aristotle is alleged to have said in his hot-selling digest *Poetics*, "for to transfer well means being able to recognize that which is related."

Well, sometimes the deft transfer of one concept to another stumbles a bit. We all have a friend who has seemed to have perfected the art of malapropos or mixed metaphor. Interesting examples can be found all across the World Wide Web. I visited a number of sites where people appear to have devoted a good portion of their waking hours to cataloging verbal blunders. Here are a few examples:

Don't bite the hand that rocks the cradle.

His dirty laundry is coming home to roost.

Frankly, we don't know whether to wind the watch or bark at the moon. (alleged to have been uttered by Dan Rather, TV newscaster)

He came out of that smelling like a bandit.

She reads like a fish out of water.

How would you feel if I were sitting in your shoes?

I don't want that monkey around my neck.

I knew that the alligators were in the swamp and that it was time to circle the wagons. (alleged to have been broadcast by **Rush Limbaugh**)

I want to be sure we don't build ourselves a bag of worms.

I'm tired of being a pawn in your lousy game of checkers!

I've got an ace up my nose.

It's right there on the tip of my brain.

She has bigger dogs to fry.

You get the idea. You don't have to know rocket surgery to do this. Metaphor is enrichment of language that can help us untangle briar patch linguistic complexities as we teach or write. It can support us as we attempt to create pure poetry, or it can startle us like a worm in the headlights. Ordinary discourse relies heavily on metaphor. Multiple connections among ideas can be crafted, and complex and exacting information can be taught or communicated in a brief phrase or two. But let the metaphorite beware. There's many a slip between the tongue and the pen.

REFERENCES

Blake, M. L. (2005). Right hemisphere syndrome. In L. L. LaPointe (Ed.), *Aphasia and related neurogenic language disorders* (3rd Ed., pp. 213–224). New York: Thieme Medical Publishers.

Botting, N. (1998). Semantic-pragmatic disorder (SPD) as a distinct diagnostic entity: Making sense of the boundaries. *International Journal of Language and Communication Disorders, 33*, 1, 87–90.

Frow, J. (2001). Metaphor and metacommunication in schizophrenic language. *Social Semiotics, 11, 3*, 275–287.

Swing, G. (2005). *Mixed Metaphors*. Retrieved April 29, 2005 from http://therussler.tripod.com/dtps/mixed_metaphors.html

CHAPTER 15

THE LONELY WHALE

It is loneliness that makes the loudest noise.

—Eric Hoffer
The True Believer, 1951

D id you hear the one about the lonely whale? What a poignant tale. The morale is ever so thinly veiled. I first heard about it in Andrew Revkin's article in the *New York Times* (Dec. 26, 2004). He entitled his story "A Song of Solitude," and it was extracted from information and data in a paper published in the December issue of *Deep Sea Research*. The original paper was published by a team of oceanographers (Watkins, Daher, George, & Rodriguez, 2004) and was dispassionately entitled "Twelve Years of Tracking 52–Hz Whale Calls from a Unique Source in the North Pacific." As Revkin comments, the story enmeshed in this esoteric research report has sparked curiosity well beyond the small circle of marine biologists who would normally pore through the technical literature on denizens of the deep. The paper reports that for over a dozen years a whale has been swimming the Pacific from central California to the Aleutian Islands. The calls of this mighty cetacean have been put on hold. Though it will call or attempt to sing, its vocalizations go unanswered. The Woods Hole Oceanographic Institution researchers have been tracking this animal since 1992 using sensitive underwater microphones. This Lonely Whale emits metronomic vocalizations at around 52 Hz (about the lowest note of a tuba), and these emissions are thought to be mating signals. So far no takers. Though the frequency (in Hz) has gradually deepened through the 1990s it is still considerably higher than the mating calls of other whale species closest to it. The giant blue and fin whales apparently have calls closer to the 52 Hz plaintive cry of Lonely Whale, but no one is responding to the isolated and pathetic calls, and it has been deprived of the socialization of the pods and swims in solitude. One of the original study's authors speculates that this whale might be congenitally malformed or miswired. Apparently it is broadcasting on the wrong frequency but receiving on the right one. Here is the ultimate example of the social isolation that can occur when one has a different voice or a defective communication system, and this has no doubt been repeated since the dawn of intraspecies ability to reach out to others like themselves.

Non-human critters communicate in interesting ways, and cetaceans such as whales and dolphins use echolocation (or sonar) as their main tool for perceiving, navigating, and communicating in the dim or murky environment where vision is not very useful. Returning sound emissions, for example regular clicks or squeaks, are processed with uncanny precision by those who use echolocation. Apparently, cetaceans can even determine the nature of their prey based on the variations in frequency that are created by differing densities of flesh and bone structure. Scientists agree that whales and other cetaceans echolocate to navigate and perceive their environment, but less consensus is reached on the mechanisms of social intraspecies communication. Interspecies communication remains controversial, however, despite the lifelong work of bio-scientists such as John Lilly to elevate communication with dolphins to something beyond a very sophisticated training paradigm.

Without meaning to anthropomorphize excessively, the lesson of the Lonely Whale seems reasonably clear. Communication is the linchpin of socialization. Communication is the glue of establishing and nurturing interpersonal relationships. Lack of communication in a society can lead to one's being ostracized or ignored. Without communication life is vapid, dry, a living death. Communication leads to understanding, to community, and to intimacy. Without tolerable communication one is destined to fail at life's three Ls: Living, Learning, and Loving, or perhaps suffer the fate of the Lonely Whale, drifting for years on the outskirts of the pod emitting pathetic and regular messages that decay and go unanswered.

That is why our mission is indispensable. We get up in the morning so we can help all those who are at risk of isolation and unwanted solitude. We yearn to help them communicate with the pod.

REFERENCES

Hoffer, E. (1951). *The true believer.* New York: Harper-Collins.

Revkin, A. C. (2004). A *song of solitude.* New York Times, Dec. 26.

Watkins, W. A., Daher, M. A., George, J. E., & Rodriguez, D. (2004). Twelve years of tracking 52-Hz whale calls from a unique source in the North Pacific. *Deep Sea Research Part 1: Oceanographic Research Papers, 51*(12) 1889–1901.

FERAL CHILDREN

Children aren't dogs; adults aren't gods.

—Haitian Proverb

One of the pleasures of attending conferences and scholarly meetings is the opportunity it affords for professional and social interaction with friends and former colleagues. A while ago I had the good fortune to present a lecture at the 5th Annual Conference on Clinical Innovations in Communication Disorders. Aside from the pleasant surrounds at James Madison University with autumn leaves coloring the vistas of the Shenandoah Valley, I met a friend of many years, Allen Boysen, who was the former head of the Audiology and Speech Pathology programs for the Department of Veterans Affairs. We had a pleasant chat about changes in our lives, mutual friends, and of course the glory days of the VA healthcare system. Then an astonishing case was brought to my attention. Boysen shared with me the details of a remarkable story of a 33-year-old man who had not developed language or other socialization skills because of a tragic and incredulous upbringing in isolation from adequate human contact. In Dr. Boysen's words, through a subsequent email:

> I had wanted to tell you a bit more about this Fiji Island male, age 33, who has primitive screeching sounds, but no meaningful verbal or nonverbal expressive communication. He was found chained to a post in a chicken yard when he was 8 years old, having lived primitively with chickens for most of his developmental years, supposedly shunned by the family for reasons not clearly discoverable. His name is xxxxx, and he is being cared for by the President of Rotary, a woman in Fiji. She engaged the interest of Linda G. who is with a documentary film company in Auckland, New Zealand. I met Linda at my granddaughter's birthday party earlier this month here in Potomac Falls, VA. Linda was visiting close friends next door. Linda asked me if I could review imaging studies and EEG results that have been collected on xxxxx to further determine whether his brain is normal enough for him to learn to communicate. By history and information from a brief videotape of his responses to a physical therapist attempting range of motion testing, it appears to me that he has petit mal seizures but . . . neurological integrity for gross motor functions, feeding, and vocalization. Otherwise, he squats and uses his hands in a prehensile pecking manner, consistent with the behavior of chickens hopping around. It sounds like someone from (a California university) has consulted on this case, but Linda could not say much about that contact. Obviously, this is a very unusual case of a human raised with animals and not communicating in any human way, even after a period of recent human contact. Do you have any thoughts about what might be done next to assess potential for language, strategies for language stimulation, and resources potentially available to support what they want to do for this young man? (A. Boysen, personal communication, October 15, 2004)

Not everyday is one consulted for an opinion on a feral child raised in relative isolation from human contact. I could offer little help other than to gather some information about other feral children and about the relative success of attempts to socialize these heartbreaking children and nurture their acquisition of human language. After researching the topic and finding a wealth of written material on the Internet and in the libraries, it became quite clear that the prognosis is as equivocal as the subject is fascinating. This essay is a bit of background on feral children, including some curious and famous cases. Much of the information in this piece has been gleaned from references and links contained on a most notable website overseen by Andrew Ward (2004). This site can be accessed at http://www.feralchildren.com/en/index.php.

Feral children, also known as wild children or wolf children, are children, who have grown up with minimal or no human contact. They are alleged to have been raised by animals (frequently by wolves) or to have somehow survived on their own. In some cases, such as in the remarkable case of the California child known as Genie, children were confined and denied normal social interaction with other people. One of the first impressions apparent from Ward's website and other sources is that there exists a rich literature on feral children. Some references classify and discuss these cases into (a) children raised by animals, (b) isolated children who lived on their own, and (c) confined children. Perhaps some of the most famous or infamous examples are those of Victor of Aveyron; Memmie LeBlanc, the Wild Girl of Champagne; and Genie, the California child of the 1970s.

David Crystal has written an intriguing entry in the *Cambridge Encyclopedia of Language* (1997) in which he lists a chronology of "children of the wild." A rich diversity of alleged circumstances, countries, and animals is apparent from the list. One of the earliest is the "Wolf child of Hesse" discovered at age 7 in the 14th Century. On the list as well is the "Bear child of Lithuania" from 1661, the "Sheep child of Ireland" from 1672, the "Pig boy of Holland" in the 1800s, the "Leopard child of India" in 1920, the "Gazelle-child of Syria" in 1946, and the "Ape child of Teheran" of 1961.

Crystal's (1997) comments about attempts to teach feral children language are particularly relevant to the readers of this journal.

> *For several hundred years, cases have been reported of children who have been reared in the wild by animals or kept isolated from all social contact. These cases are listed below, adapted from Lucien Malson's* Wolf Children. ... *Sometimes the information is based on little more than a brief press report. At other times, the cases have been studied in detail—in particular, the stories of Victor, ... and Genie. (p. 148)*

Crystal also reported the rather dubious experiments of an ancient Egyptian king (Psamtik I) who in the 7th century presented two newborn infants to the care of shepherds, with the instructions that they should not be taught to speak in order to observe which language they spoke first, which would then be regarded as the world's oldest language. Crystal stated that the reports about the children's language abilities created a clear picture (Crystal clear?), that the children could not speak at all and had no comprehension of language.

Efforts to teach other feral children to speak were met with similar frustration. Crystal stated that most attempts to teach wild children language failed. Some are reported to have learned some speech, and Tomko of Hungary in 1767 was reputed to have learned both Slovak and German, but little evidence is presented to verify these reports. Two Indian children are said to have learned some sign language. The famous Victor, the "Wild Boy of Averyon," remained unable to speak, though it is said he could understand and say *"lait"* (milk) and *"O Dieu"* (Oh God). Victor also was reported to have learned to read a number of words. Crystal reports the two most successful cases on record of speech acquisition are that of Kaspar Hauser, whose speech is reported to have been quite "advanced," and Genie, the famous and heartrending girl of the 1970s who learned a few words immediately after her discovery and whose progress was considerable until the roadblock of syntax was encountered.

Genie turned out to be a rich "forbidden experiment" for a team of scientists and linguists. This young girl was discovered in a Los Angeles home on November 4, 1970. She was a lifelong victim of bizarre child abuse and isolation. On her discovery at age 13 years, 7 months, she was tied to a potty chair. She had no language skills and would only babble like an infant. It is reported that she was probably beaten for attempting to vocalize or make noise. For over a decade she had been completely restrained. When released for the first time, Genie's motoric behavior was described as a strange "bunny walk" holding her hands in front of her and hopping and clawing. Genie engendered a lot of research attention and funding, and her progress was followed and reported by a crossdisciplinary team of scientists. Although initially showing great progress, she eventually plateaued in her language acquisition. Language structure and syntax were much more taxing to her than merely learning vocabulary items. Even after much training and exposure to a natural societal and linguistic environment, she stumbled with word order and the grammar of language. She never became adept at phrases and sentences and got only as far as using phrases such as "applesauce buy store." Great debate ensued as to whether or not Genie had passed what Lenneberg (1967) had described as the "Critical Age Hypothesis," which held that a crucial window of opportunity existed for the development of language. Others argued that perhaps Genie's brain was missing something that was crucial to learning syntax and more advanced forms of language.

Susan Curtiss has written a comprehensive compilation of the language intervention attempts with Genie in her book entitled *Genie: A Psycholinguistic Study of a Modern-Day "Wild Child" (Perspectives in neurolinguistics and psycholinguistics)* (Curtiss, 1977). The literature is replete with linguistic and behavioral writings on Genie, and one can access the Communication Disorders Dome, PubMed, or even Google to find extensive information on the attempts to nurture Genie's language and social development. In the late 1970s, Genie's mother prevented the Genie Team from having contact with Genie. Although Genie lived with her mother after her discovery, it is reported that her mother was unable to care for her, and in subsequent years Genie reportedly has been in a series of foster homes.

Feral children are also a rich subject for hoaxes and exploitation by the popular media. Films and popular culture books have been written about Genie and other children. Some have blurred the line between sensational case reporting and fiction. One classic example listed on Ward's website, un-der "Hoaxes," is that of the Wild Boy of Burundi. The *Johannesburg Times* carried the first article about a young boy who allegedly was raised by a band of monkeys. Harlan Lane, a scientist who had a long interest in feral children had just published a book about Victor, the Wild Boy of Aveyron. Lane and colleague Richard Pillard, a psychiatrist from Boston University, set out to investigate the Burundi feral child report. Their investigation revealed that the boy had never lived with monkeys. Instead, he was determined to be severely autistic, that his mother died in childbirth, and the father died in civil unrest. The boy's identity was apparently lost, and he was passed among various agencies and foster homes. Lane has written an account of this hoax in a book entitled *The Wild Boy of Burundi: A Study of an Outcast Child* (Lane, 1978).

Ward reports other apparent hoaxes including that of the Syrian Gazelle Boy who was alleged to have been found running naked with a pack of ga-zelles in the desert. Photographs of him with a blatantly obvious "farmer's tan" lend credence to Ward's report that this case was a hoax perpetrated by bored newspaper reporters stuck in the middle of the desert and eager for some sensational copy. Another case report with subsequent confes-sion that it was a hoax is that of the "Nullarbor Nymph," a 17-year-old girl who was alleged to be living with a mob of kangaroos in Western Australia. This story was eventually revealed as a publicity stunt conceived to play a practical joke on tourists.

Despite the hoaxes and the sensationalism surrounding many of the re-ported cases of feral children, there is no doubt that a tragic and valid history of isolated, confined, and feral children exists. These unfortunate circumstances offer the opportunity for "forbidden experiments," particularly on the weighty issues of genetic versus environmental influences on language acquisition and socialization. The nature-nurture argument will be with us for decades to come, no doubt, but perhaps the remarkable stories of the Fijian boy alleg-edly raised with chickens, and the heartbreak of Victor and Genie, will help us learn more about the significant and complex enigma of brain versus envi-ronment. The old Haitian proverb at the beginning of this essay aptly relates to feral children. Surely children are not dogs, and the morally impoverished adults who allow these catastrophes to happen are far from gods.

REFERENCES

Crystal, D. (1997). *Cambridge encyclopedia of language.* Cambridge: Cambridge University Press.

Curtiss, S. (1977). *Genie: A psycholinguistic study of a modern-day "wild child" (Perspectives in neurolinguistics and psycholinguistics).* New York: Academic Press.

Lane, H. (1978). *The wild boy of Burundi: A study of an outcast child.* (New York: Random House).

Lenneberg, E. (1967). *Biological foundations of language.* New York: John Wiley & Sons.

Ward, A. (2004). FeralChildren.com. Retrieved October 27, 2004, from http://www.feralchildren.com/en/index.php

CHAPTER 17

BIOLOGY OF HOPE

We can be sure that the greatest hope for maintaining equilibrium in the face of any situation rests within ourselves.

—Francis J. Braceland, *O Magazine*, April 2003

True hope is swift, and flies with swallow's wings.

—W. Shakespeare, *King Richard III*, Act V, Scene 2

I hope I'm not repeating myself. I hope I'm not repeating myself. I get the faint smell of déjà vu vis-à-vis the topic of hope, optimism, and its relationship to wellness. I recall sometime in the recent past on these pages of characterizing the optimist as always seeing the donut and the pessimist as always seeing the hole. Trite, but half true. These days the topic of dispositional optimism, hope, if you will, is much in the writings of the social psychology of health care. The range of conviction about the healing power of hope is wide. This range spills over and muddies the boundaries of science and belief; and so any pronouncement on the topic necessarily must tiptoe through the two lips and attempt to define clearly the position of the pronouncer. I stand firmly in the middle. The quotations from those who have made odds-defying recoveries are filled with suggestions that others, too, would recover and achieve miracles if only they would believe, pray, or never become pessimistic. The data set is remarkably free of evidence from those who did believe, pray, and embrace optimism and still didn't make it. I am always amazed at the reasoning of those who have survived some horrendous tragedy, such as a plane crash in the Everglades or a sunken ferry off the coast of Bangladesh, who are quoted as saying that a divine power smiled on them because of their deep faith or belief. What about the others with the same beliefs who did not survive? It makes one wonder about attribution; cause and effect; and the nether world of the role of belief; faith, optimism, and hope on wellness and life quality.

For years the influence of mind on body was viewed as scientifically disreputable, sullied by charlatans and quacks. Practitioners and gurus of alternative or "complementary" medicine traditionally have been more aligned with entrepreneurial belief mongers than with empirical scientists. Month after month, the pages of literary works such as *Skeptical Inquirer* are filled with debunking articles of junk science applied to healing. But soft, now comes a new direction. As our bard reminds us, "true hope is swift," and may be gaining some scientific respectability.

The biology of hope has been an alluring topic recently, and credible scientists are laboring in clinics and laboratories across the globe trying to unlock the secrets of the interactions of mind and body. Recent writings about optimism, wellness, and the biology of hope are beginning to tie philosophical and theoretical discussions to empirical research of dispositional optimism as an individual difference that might have a reliable beneficial link to good mood, perseverance, achievement, and certain aspects of physical health (Peterson, 2000). Surely many uncertainties remain, but as in all precise trailblazing, each conclusion or confirmation raises a nest of questions waiting to be pursued. Such is the process of scientific inquiry. Major questions loom about optimism as a research topic and as a societal value. As one wag once remarked, "How come we're optimistic, when we're all going to die?" Well the answer is firmly entrenched in quality of life. Whether you share the life expectancy of a fruit fly, a Fiji green-banded lizard, a farmer from South Dakota, or an Eastern Orthodox nun from Tbilisi, you still share the inherent and noble goal of living life optimally, be it a matter of hours or decades. And life quality and wellness may be directly linked to biological changes brought about by state of mind, particularly hope and optimism.

A recent study of cardiac patients in Miami investigated independent and mediated contributions of personality, coping, social support, and depressive symptoms to physical functional outcomes among patients in rehabilitation (Shen, McCreary, & Myers, 2004). These researchers found that optimism and social support contribute to health outcomes not only directly, but indirectly through the mediation of less engagement in detrimental coping. In another study of hope in participants with chronic disease, optimistic chronically ill patients did not have biased and unrealistic perceptions of their health status, and the existence of positive efficacy expectancies appeared to encourage beneficial self-care behaviors (DeRidder, Fournier, & Bensing, 2004).

We are barely on the threshold of developing a firm scientific understanding of many psychosocial elements important to mind-body relationships. We must continue to discard the chaff and the detritus of poorly conceived wellness psycho-bunk espoused and sold by charlatans and shamans and discover those mind states that truly and reliably change body states. Then we will have something, and the biology of hope will find that equilibrium that rests within ourselves and flies with swallow's wings.

REFERENCES

DeRidder, D., Fournier, M., & Bensing, J. (2004). Does optimism affect symptom report in chronic disease?: What are its consequences for self-care behavior and physical functioning? *Journal of Psychosomatic Research, 56*(3), 341–350.

Peterson, C. (2000). The future of optimism. *American Psychologist, 55*(1), 44–55.

Shen, B., McCreary, C., & Myers, H. (2004). Independent and mediated contributions of personality, coping, social support, and depressive symptoms to physical functioning outcome among patients in cardiac rehabilitation. *Journal of Behavioral Medicine, 27*(1), 19–62.

CHAPTER 18

DREAMS

Dreaming permits each and every one of us to be quietly and safely insane every night of our lives.

—Charles William Dement

Follow your dream. Unless it's the one where you're at work in your underwear during a fire drill.

—Zadok Rabinowitz

L inguistic conundrums abound with the word *dream*. Did you dream you would reach your dream? The quotations above attest to the polysemantic notion of *dream*. It can be an objective or an aspiration, or it can be the insanity or sweet oblivion of our sleep state. Those nightly visitors that cavort between states of consciousness and unconsciousness have been a source of wonder and inscrutability as long as humankind has recorded experience. Caves in France and at other anthropological sites show pictographs believed to depict dream states. We spend a third of our lives sleeping, but the enchanted loom in our brain never slumbers. Yet the purpose and nature of dreaming remains one of science's great unsolved mysteries. No wonder it is fertile ground for charlatans, quacks, interpreters, and the twilight zone of voodoo science and junk research. No wonder that Freud had to be reminded that sometimes a cigar is just a cigar. Not everything that is known about dreams is bunk, however. Cognitive scientists in sleep disorders clinics and laboratories around the world are piecing together theories of sleep and tantalizing hypotheses about dreaming. Even a cursory venture through the publications of these laboratories reveals that there are many evidence-based truisms about sleep and dreaming. For example:

- Most dreaming takes place during Rapid Eye Movement (REM) sleep.
- Dreaming seems necessary for good health. When people are deprived of REM sleep, they have difficulty with normal daily activities and may hallucinate.
- People spend about 1½ hours a night dreaming and have a mean of about 1,000 dreams a year, even if many of them are not recalled.
- Dreamers have four to six separate dreams each night, but the last dream is usually the one recalled.
- Dreams that occur during the same sleep cycle usually are variations on the same topic or theme.
- Dream recall varies widely across participants in sleep studies. Some people remember a dream every night and others cannot report recall of a single dream over a span of several months.
- Most dream rememberers report dream recall three or four nights per week.
- Neither sleep quality nor length of sleep appears to be associated with dream recall.
- Creativity and problem solving have long been anecdotally related to dreaming ("The answer came to me in a dream." Keith Richards dreamed the guitar riff in the song *I Can't Get No Satisfaction* and on awakening proceeded to record it), and recent empirical research seems to provide some evidence for the revelatory potential of dreams.

Many of the findings just listed are widely available in review papers on sleep and dreams, but a couple of the more intriguing connections between personality type and dreams or creativity and dreaming have been spurred on by the results of two recent studies (Wagner, Grais, Haider, Verleger, & Born, 2004; Watson, 2003).

The study by Wagner et al. (2004) is from a Neuroendrocrinology Laboratory in Germany and was published in the journal *Nature* by a research team led by scientist Jan Born. In one of those scientific news-feeding frenzies, it was picked up by wire services and distributed across the world by print and broadcast media. The study has sparked debate and a good deal of public interest in the topic of dreams and creativity and problem solving. In the study, volunteers who had 8 hours of sleep were three times more likely than sleep-deprived participants to figure out a hidden rule solution to a mathematics test. Other researchers have long thought or reported anecdotes about problem solving or creativity occurring in dreams or after sleep, but the German team designed a clever experiment to offer evidence on their hypotheses. The implications are obvious and far-reaching. Seventy million people in the United States suffer from sleep deprivation that may contribute to accidents, health problems, and degraded behavioral and academic performance. The old strategy of "pulling an allnighter" and cramming for academic tests may be contraindicated, and in fact may prevent information consolidation presumed to occur during dreaming and a good night's sleep. "Get a good night's sleep" may replace the time-honored advice of "Cram it. Damn it. Take the test and slam it."

Dream behavior always has provoked a pervasive popular interest. Cyberspace is alive with dream gurus, dream doctors, and New Age interpreters of our sleep netherworld. There are associations and societies both scientific and quasiscientific that offer opinion, advice, interpretations, and occasionally some peer-reviewed evidence on dream behavior. One of the interesting topics to peruse is the commonality of certain recurring themes in reported dreams. Popular recurring dream themes include:

- Falls, falling, airborne behavior
- Being chased with inept attempts at escape
- Turbulent, near-miss, under-the-wires airplane rides and landings (one of my recurring themes)
- Missing the final exam, or showing up for the final exam after not having attended class the entire term (another of my recurring dreams and reported fairly commonly among people who have had extended academic experience)
- Bird and animal attacks (wrestling the python, so to speak, and fending off the seagulls)
- Return of deceased loved ones
- Public humiliation and nudity at public appearances
- Shattered teeth, loose incisors, or teeth falling out
- Catastrophes such as nuclear holocaust, tornadoes on the horizon, or hurricanes bearing down

- Finding gold, hidden treasure, or an ice-cream tree
- Being able to walk or breathe underwater

The list of common recurring dream themes seems more like a nightmare list to me, but therein lies the fascination of attempts to sort out meaning, interpretation, or the linkage of dream matter to personality or to current worries and stress. No doubt cognitive and neuroscientists, perhaps some of those counted among our readership, will continue to unravel the tangles of memory consolidation and meaning in these nightly dreamscapes and help us achieve a more empirical understanding of these universal and mystifying phenomena. In the meantime, take this issue of bedside reading material with you as you settle down for another cycle of restitution, stress resolution, creativity, and informational problem solving. Enjoy the quiet safety of another night of insanity. Sweet dreams.

REFERENCES

Wagner, U., Gais, S., Haider, H., Verleger, R., & Born, J. (2004). Sleep inspires insight. *Nature, 427,* 352–355.

Watson, D. (2003). To dream, perchance to remember: Individual differences in dream recall. *Journal of Personality and Individual Differences, 34*(7), 1271–1286.

CHAPTER 19

A Little Night
Tafelspitz

... When I am, as it were, completely myself, entirely alone, and of good cheer—say traveling in a carriage, or walking after a good meal, or during the night when I cannot sleep—it is on such occasions that my ideas flow best, and most abundantly. Whence and how they come, I know not, nor can I force them.

—Wolfgang Amadeus Mozart (1756–1791)

So from whence and how do ideas come? The origin of creativity puzzled Wolfgang even as it does contemporary neurocognitive scientists. Perhaps there are conditions that set the muse. But the muse is notoriously fickle and can arrive and evaporate prior to fruition. Mozart's prodigious output—more than 600 works—including instrumental combinations, concertos, vocal works, and operas are ample evidence that even as a child he possessed a thorough domination of the technical resources of musical composition as well as a wondrous imagination. But the font of ideas needed priming, even for one of the great geniuses of civilization. Mozart knew that ideas could not be forced, but must be nurtured, coaxed, and bathed in the proper ambience to be born.

The proper ambience for some recent creativity for aphasiologists proved to be the very streets that once carried the clip-clop carriages of Mozart, Hayden, Schubert, and several Strausses (Strice?). The magnificent Austrian Academy of Sciences building on Dr. Ignaz Seipel-Platz in Vienna, Austria was the site of the 41st annual meeting of the Academy of Aphasia, an organization of neurologists, neurolinguists, neuropsychologists, and speech-language pathologists who have a particular curiosity about the enigma of aphasia. Arthur Koestler is alleged to have once said that creativity is a learning process where the teacher and pupil are located in the same individual. Here in Vienna in October of 2003 was the prime opportunity to once again fuse teacher and pupil. The proper broth for the *Tafelspitz* of creativity during these Viennese autumn days proved to be the chance once again to present, interact, react, and socialize with some of the leading thinkers in the world of aphasiology. Dr. Jacqueline Stark, an American who has lived in Austria for 30 years, took command of the local arrangements and provided an elegant and efficient site for this meeting of minds. The cherubs and frescoes of the building were commented upon and put into historical perspective by Professor Wolfgang Dressler of the Austrian Academy of Sciences, and then the program was turned over to the scientists and clinicians who had traveled from Australia, Hong Kong, Canada, the United States, Japan, and all parts of Europe. Papers, symposia, and posters covered such topics as language deficits and basal ganglia lesions; lexical organization as revealed by intracarotid sodium amytal injection; intrasubject variability of cognition and word retrieval; semantic priming in Parkinson disease; the Jackson versus Broca debate of 1868; and impact of resources restriction on processing non-literal utterances. The Academy luncheon speaker was Professor Dr. Claus Wallesch from Germany who presented a historical treatise on Freud as an aphasiologist.

So how has this conference in this city of museums, music, *fiakers*, Sacher torte, huge *weiner schnitzels*, and *tafelspitz* (boiled beef) contributed to some semblance of creativity and carryover to our mundane practices and routine daily responsibilities? I can only speak for one attendant. I was enlightened by interactions with colleagues such as Bruce Murdoch, Malcolm McNeil, Heinz Karl Stark, Tim Shallice, Helen Chenery, Steven Small, Jacqui Laures, Subhash Bhatnagar, Sam Po Law, and Yves Joanette, among others. The scientific interactions at both the papers and the social events generated ideas and germinated a few seeds that were long dormant. One practical outcome was the initiation of several ideas on how to improve the design of a study we are currently wrestling with on the effects of semantic distraction on word retrieval and recognition in aphasia. A wonderful presentation by Crutch and Warrington from London elicited ways of resolving determination of semantic relatedness on stimuli to be presented for processing by people with aphasia. Those ideas will be articulated at our laboratory meeting in approximately one hour from the writing of these words with the fondest hope that our dilemma of semantic relatedness will be addressed and solved.

And so it goes with the ambiance that nurtures creativity, or at the very least the resolution of sticky problems. Mozart knew not from whence or how the ideas sprung forth, but he did realize that under particular conditions, ideas flow best. His death at age 35 is surrounded in controversy, but one of the theories advanced is that the genius died of a cerebral hemorrhage, one of the very causes of aphasia that this august group came to Vienna to discuss (Baroni, 1997).

Thank you, colleagues at the Academy of Aphasia in the glorious city of Vienna for once again being catalytic. Sometimes a little night music or the sleeplessness from a bit too much *tafelspitz* can rouse the muse.

May you find some ideas in the muse-aic of contributions in this quarter's journal as well.

REFERENCE

Baroni, C. (1997). The pathobiography and death of Wolfgang Amadeus Mozart: From legend to reality. *Human Pathology, 28*(5), 519–521.

CHAPTER 20

WHALES, BRAINS, AND ISLANDS

. . . for no man lives in the external truth among salts and acids, but in the warm, phantasmagoric chamber of his brain, with the painted windows and the storied wall.

—Robert Louis Stevenson (1850–1894)

M r. Stevenson had a way with words. For in the phantasmagoric chamber we entrap all of the treasured islands of mystery and history. I just read a review, written by John J. Puccio, of the DVD of the 1950 Disney classic kid adventure movie *Treasure Island*, and it struck a chord of familiarity and remembrance about this great yarn of sea life, pirates, buried gold, and an ensemble of creepy characters. As with Puccio, I think Stevenson's book version was one of the first novels I ever read cover to cover. What a troupe of rascals, all of whom were brought brilliantly to life by the cast of the 1950's film. Bobby Driscoll was the Disney ultracute young Jim Hawkins, thrown into a plot of mayhem and mutiny and surrounded by Blind Pew, Billy Bones, Black Dog, Captain Smollett, the scraggy castaway Ben Gunn, and the archetypal menacing pirate Long John Silver (played brilliantly enough to trigger a hundred nightmares by Robert Newton). Long John Silver launched a thousand pirate impersonators and a string of fast food fish and chips stores with his parrot, wooden peg leg ("all natural lower extremity prosthesis" in today's language), and model pirate utterance, "aaarrrgh."

The book and the 1950's movie are enduring classics embedded in our warm brain vaults. The frequent film remakes (e.g., Muppet version as well as the latest outer space computer-animated version *Treasure Planet*) don't come close to the benchmark by which all children's adventure yarns are measured, or to the print version, which takes ever so perfect advantage of the theater of the mind. It's on DVD with lots of extra scenes, so run out to your local memory depository shop and rent a return to yesterday.

All of this may have been triggered by a recent voyage to another island, filled, as it were, with treasures of its own. This year's Clinical Aphasiology Conference was held on Orcas Island in the Puget Sound off the coast of the state of Washington. We enjoyed a marvelous program, with a symposium and entire section on the theme of model-based aphasia treatment. David Plaut, from Carnegie-Mellon University, engaged us with computational modeling of language processing along with advances in computational lesions and predictions of recovery. Thanks to a grant from the NIDCD, a division of the National Institutes of Health, this year's conference program chair Argye B. Hillis and grant coordinator Connie Tompkins were able to infuse the program with special topics, keynote speakers and commentators, and young ideas. A number of doctoral students were funded to participate in this mentored conference experience. In the words of one of the silverbacks who has attended nearly all of the 30 some years of the Clinical Aphasiology Conference, "It is refreshing to see that the torch will be passed to such impressive, bright, young scholars."

In addition to special sessions, the conference once again enjoyed the enduring tenets and features of this annual meeting:

1. The location must be at a desirable destination resort.
2. There must be as much program time allowed for discussion and questions as there is for formal presentation.

3. Activities must be planned that allow participants to network, communicate informally, eat together, socialize, and exchange ideas on clinical aspects of aphasiology.

4. The program and interchanges must show scholarly rigor, but with a civilized and collegial tone rather than academic clawing and neckbiting.

These features of the Clinical Aphasiology Conference endear it to those of us who have attended over 30 of them (see the CAC website at http:// www.clinicalaphasiology.org/). Particularly notable this year was the chance to enjoy the natural beauty of the Northwestern United States and the island life of the Puget Sound. We saw pods of orca whales, sea otters, sea lions, several majestic American bald eagles, and an albino deer. We enjoyed the views of the archipelago from the top of Mt. Constitution, and we experienced sea kayaking, sailing, marvelous art galleries, Copper River wild salmon, and sloshed cold beer with world class Penn Cove Mussels. Margaret Rogers and her most competent crew of local arrangements people vanned, ferried, and coddled participants with red licorice twizzlers, orange juice, sunshine, and gracious Northwest hospitality and good humor.

All of these ingredients make for an enriched experience. Working daily with people who face the challenge of damaged brains and lost language, memory, and self is a daunting task, but it is enriched by experiences of whales, islands, and vivid professional interaction. As Mr. Stevenson suggested, the warm chamber of the brain stores all of this mystery. We shall continue our daily grind to understand it and crack the secrets of this treasured island. But we mustn't forget to get out of the salts and the acids now and then to check up on the pirates.

Enjoy the voyage and enjoy this issue of *JMSLP*. Aaarrgh.

CHAPTER 21

TIME AFTER TIME

Time is the coin of your life. It is the only coin you have, and only you can determine how it will be spent. Be careful lest you let other people spend it for you.

—Carl Sandburg (1878–1967)

W hat time is it? Late again. Late again. Eight o'clock. Nine o'clock. Quarter to ten. Time is precious. Time is money. Time is what we have. Time is what we are. We organize it and it keeps us on track. Do we control it or does it control us? It allows us to scratch things off our to-do list and accomplish. *Accomplish* has some interesting synonyms in the old Microsoft thesaurus. *Achieve. Do. Get done. Complete. Finish. Bring about. Pull off. Undertake.* Time is a healer, but may not be as good a beautician. Time flies. Time is an illusion. Time wounds all heels.

Time can be cruel and oppressive. It is a powerful dictator. It tells us where to go and when to go there. We work ourselves into a sweat against the press of appointments, deadlines, and an insidious attitude of urgency. Life in the new century and in our "civilized" culture converts to a daily grind of struggle against the clock. And clocks are everywhere. In our pocket. On our wrists. In our cars. On our palm pilots. On our walls and ovens and coffee pots and CD players. Is it surprising that we have evolved (or mutated) into over-booked, appointment addicted, overwhelmed drones? Like Svengali's Trilby we shuffle along in a hypnotic dedication to our electronic masters.

Jay Walljasper and his editorial staff have written a biting feature in the *Utne Reader* (Walljasper, 2003) on the domination of our appointment books and how to cope with smothering time pressure. They have some interesting and worthy suggestions for expanding time, resisting the urge to over-schedule, and for returning to the more natural rhythms so we can let life, not the clock, decree our every move. As Walljasper and his colleagues point out, on the job, at school, and at home people all over the globe have become virtual slaves to their schedules. Our tramping is charted for us, many times in precise quarter hour allocations, on our desk calendars and Day-at-a-Glance diaries. Some feel we are no longer in control. We are not leading our lives, but merely following a vertiginous timetable of duties, commitments, meetings, dead-lines, and booked-in "leisure" activities.

The emerging blitz of new technology has promised to liberate us, to save precious time. Instead it has cranked up our daily life tempo with cell phone, palm organizer, and e-mail expectations of on-the-spot response and action. We are never out of contact, even when we are supposedly out of contact. Our vacations and holidays are not sacrosanct anymore, and we are connected on vacation in Fiji or at the fishing cottage in New Brunswick. If we are never disconnected or out of the loop, are we ever not working? Magic moments and the succor of spontaneity are all but dead. Is this healthful? Can you hear me now? And where is all that time we're supposedly saving?

My friend Bruce Murdoch at the University of Queensland, Australia, told me of an interesting survey that was conducted at a major Western university that tallied the traditional productivity of researchers and academics (number of grants, publications, presentations). A sample was drawn from across disciplines from the precomputer era (a block of years in the late 1970s and 80s) and contrasted with productivity of the same researchers and same disciplines in the postcomputer, time-saving era of the late 1990s. No significant differences were found in the amount of productivity across the two blocks of time. Although this survey is only anecdotal it is perhaps not surprising since, just as nature abhors a vacuum, time when saved is flooded with more tasks, and perchance not the tasks that result in more traditional scholarly productivity.

The *Utne Reader* group has some marvelous ideas and tips on how to stop, shift, and expand time. As Rechtschaffen (2003) writes in the January–February issue (pp. 63–64), nearly everyone responds negatively to the query "Do you have enough time in your life?" Even prisoners "doing time" were so heavily scheduled and regimented that they said they had no time. So it's high time those of us who feel that way did something about it. The *Utne* gang presents the following sane approaches.

- Find quick, easy ways to break your demanding tempo
  Learn to pause and take a deep breath when booting up your computer. Don't jump on the first ring of the phone but let it go a few rings. The simple act of pausing can interrupt the hectic rhythm and at least create the illusion of expanding time.

- Create time boundaries
  These are oases of time for ourselves. Perhaps stopping at the Sweet Shoppe and getting a cup of latte and strolling more leisurely from the parking lot to the office will do it. Set aside 15 minutes to read something you wouldn't normally have time for, preferably some escape, popcorn literature. Listen to a great accordion sonata. Pick up the threads of your childhood. Break up your day by closing your office door for 15 minutes and engaging in contemplation or meditation that is uninterrupted. Perhaps you might even go so far as contemplating your navel or even measuring the depth of your navel. This, however, is not recommended if there is any risk of anyone entering unannounced.

- Honor the mundane
  Instead of thinking about what to do next, enjoy the process of whatever ordinary activity needs to be done. Enjoy the rich textures and flavor of the Halibut *Court Bullion* you are eating instead of thinking about what to do next. Take a walk and spot two new bugs or plants instead of hustling to finish up your obsessive exercise time. Notice the cool side of the pillow.

- Create spontaneous time
  Block out some time for spontaneity. This may seem oxymoronic, but if we set aside some of our future and just go somewhere with no particular destination in mind we may stumble into impulsivity that rewards us. Rechtschaffen suggests picking out an afternoon 3 weeks from now, writing your own name into your appointment book, and leaving work early for an unplanned jaunt. Watch some kids play soccer. Go to Tom Brown Park and be surprised by the vibrant music and dancing of an African group picnic.

- Create time retreats
  Go somewhere that breaks the rhythms and tempos of your ordinary moments. Watch and listen to some minutes going by that are unfilled with planned activities. Find a spot to be still. Play dead. Don't frighten your family, but let yourself drift into beta. Let the time block be variable so that you are controlling time and not vice versa.

So find some time to read this issue of *JMSLP*. We have another resonant compilation of offerings. The Academy of Neurological Communication Disorders and Sciences (ANCDS) committees continue their work on the development of practice guidelines, and in this issue we have an update as well as fully developed guidelines for direct attention training. We also present an article on electropalatographic (EPG) assessment of dysarthria in traumatic brain injury by the excellent research group at the University of Queensland's Motor Speech Research Unit. From the Mayo Clinic in the United States comes an article on speech-language disorders in corticobasal degeneration. We have as well a clinical report on communication in epilepsy and some normative data on a frequently used measure of information processing.

I hope you find time to peruse our journal and check off the important things on your to-do list. People have puzzled how to manage time successfully since time immemorial. I wish you success in coping with increasing time demands. For time is of the essence. As the American baseball player was alleged to have said when asked for the time, "Do you mean now?" So be careful with your now. Be careful with time, the coin of your life. Spend it wisely and don't let it spend you.

REFERENCES

Rechtschaffen, S. (2003). How to expand time. *Utne Reader,* Jan–Feb, pp. 63–64.

Walljasper, J. (2003). Our schedules, our selves. *Utne Reader,* Jan–Feb, pp. 61–63.

CHAPTER 22

MOXON AND THE FLYING TRAPEZE

Who knows only his own generation remains always a child.

—George Norlin (1939)

W here were you in 1866? Do you remember it as a pivotal year? Ah, the good times? Ah, the music. The explosive discoveries. Alfred Nobel, the Swedish chemist, invented dynamite and was to lend his name to one of the most prestigious foundations worldwide. It would undertake the task of recognizing accomplishments in physics, chemistry, physiology and medicine, and literature. Perhaps the most notable of the annually awarded honors is to the person recognized as deserving the Nobel Peace Prize. It would be nice to be around when the ideals of the recipients of the peace prize are realized. Given the human limbic system and current events, it may be a diaphanous goal.

Ironically, H. G. Wells, the British author who penned *War of the Worlds*, was born in 1866 as well, and Dostoevsky published *Crime and Punishment*. In France, Degas began to paint his lovely ballet scenes, and Charles Baudelaire was cranking out risqué stories and poems. In the United States and Europe, teenagers were dancing and humming along to such 1866 music as *The Man on the Flying Trapeze, When You and I were Young, Maggie*, and the ever popular *Father's a Drunkard and Mother is Dead*.

Of course, 1866 was a banner year for continued debate and discussion of the intellectual hot topics of brain and language. Just 3 years earlier Paul Broca had shaken up the Societe d' Anthropologie of Paris by presenting his cases associating the left frontal lobe with the "seat of articulate speech." Although Broca and Wernicke are the 19th-century celebrities associated with brain and language behavior, another and lesser known writer on the topic was recently brought to my attention. At one of the convivial coffees at the American Speech-Language-Hearing Association annual meeting in Atlanta, I had the pleasure of visiting with a long-time friend and colleague, Dr. Hugh Buckingham from Louisiana State University. We reminisced about our overlap days in Gainesville, Florida, where Hugh would grace our Friday patient review and disposition meetings and offer insights and observations of a psycholinguistic slant. It was always instructive and most often entertaining from a researcher who can speak fluent jargon aphasia in several languages. At our Atlanta meeting, Dr. Buckingham told me about an interesting 1866 article he had just read by W. Moxon, M.D., Pathologist and Curator of the Museum at Guy's Hospital in London.

Moxon's article, "On the Connection between Loss of Speech and Paralysis of the Right Side," was published in *The British and Foreign Medico-Chirurgical Review*, Volume XXXVII, January–April, 1866, 481–489. In it, Moxon waxes enthusiastically about the recent revelations of Broca. Moxon also interprets and extends some ideas about language and "mental science" and reveals some remarkably sophisticated views on higher cortical function and cerebral asymmetry. Says Moxon:

> It is, I think, not over venturesome to say, that no observations have for many years excited in the medical world more intense and general interest than those of M. Broca, upon the coincidence of loss of speech with paralysis of the right side, which have been brought before the profession in England by Dr. H. Jackson, in a comprehensive and able record of cases. (p. 481)

Moxon proceeds to discuss concepts related to the "astonishing" loss of speech and language in "bilaterally symmetrical" organs of speech from "unilateral disease."

Moxon constructs intriguing examples reminiscent of autostimulation to illustrate some of his points. A careful reading reveals some insightful observations about divided attention, a concept that plays an increasing role in theories of cognitive resource allocation and aphasia, as well as on the relationship of attention to memory. He also, as Buckingham has observed, has a good deal to say about the nature of disruption of volitional movements that might be related to contemporary theories of apraxia. Moxon says,

> *I would first notice, how very difficult it is to make one's hands execute opposite motions at the same time; let any one, as Dr. Carpenter says, try to make one hand revolve in one direction whilst the other revolves in the opposite direction, and he will experience this difficulty.*

> *Now let any one try to make them both revolve at the same time in the same direction, and it will be evidently the most natural thing in the world . . .*

> *In learning to play upon the piano, a very long time is taken before the learner becomes able to give his attention to the hands separately, so as to make them perform different parts simultaneously . . .*

> *To view it in another way: the difference of facility with like and opposite simultaneous motions, is a measure of the degree of attention saved to the hand which follows its fellow . . .*

> *. . . memory being only the mark left in the brain by former acts of attention, being that which persists of former attention . . .*

> *. . . in ordinary speech the word or even the part of a sentence to which we are accustomed, comes to the tongue without the attention of the mind to the particular movements required, and often with an inappreciably low degree of attention to the word or sentence, as when long strings of sentences are muttered unconsciously by one absent in mind. (pp. 485 and 487)*

Moxon advanced some most interesting 19th-century interpretations and concepts about topics that even in this day are incompletely understood and continue to cause consternation in our late-night private thoughts: asymmetry and bilateralism in higher cortical function; the relationship of speech and language; the peculiar harmony of the left and right cortical hemispheres in linguistic function; the role of attention in memory and in language acquisition and use; the peculiar cognitive domains that play a role in linguistic breakdown; the role of loss of memory for movement in apraxia and other movement disorders. These are issues that may still be incompletely understood and explained even in 2066. We can learn however by learning from previous generations. Thank you Dr. Buckingham for sharing your discovery of Moxon, a lesser recognized 19th-century neuro-thinker.

The quotation on the portal of the Norlin Library at the University of Colorado on the risks of knowing your own generation is as relevant today as when it was inscribed in 1939. Let's hope we continue to find previously veiled bits of wisdom such as that advanced by Moxon as he hummed along to *The Man on the Flying Trapeze.*

REFERENCE

Moxon, W. (1866). On the connexion (sic) between loss of speech and paralysis of the right side. *The British and Foreign Medico-Chirurgical Review,* Vol. XXXVII, January–April, 481–489.

CHAPTER 23

SUSHI, GATOR TAIL, AND KNEE BANJOS

I came from old Osaka, with a banjo on my knee.

—Anon

Sometimes things get a little lost in translation. Perhaps one of the most classic translation blooper legends involves the report that when Coca-Cola was first sold in China it was given a similar phonetically based name; but the characters used for the name allegedly meant "Bite the wax tadpole."

Other international corporations have stumbled as well. Bacardi marketed a fruity drink with the name *Pavian* to suggest French chic, but *Pavian* apparently means "baboon" in German. A Swedish convenience store named *Servus* discovered that their minor problem with Hungarian shoplifters could be traced to the translation of *Servus* as "yours for free" in Hungarian. Chevrolet's marketing of the Chevrolet Nova in South America ran into some sales resistance that may have been related to the fact that *no va* in Spanish means "doesn't go." An American t-shirt maker in Miami printed shirts for the Spanish market that promoted the Pope's visit. Instead of the desired "I Saw the Pope" in Spanish, the shirts proclaimed "I Saw the Potato."

We recently had our own experience with translation idiosyncrasies during a visit here at Florida State University by a contingent of professionals in health care from Japan, headed by Dr. Isami Kumakura of the Kawasaki University of Medical Welfare. Dr. Keiichi Takeda, of the Osaka University of Education, has coordinated previous exchanges. The expertise of this group's translator, Kayoko Shigamatsu ensured that our lectures were translated with amazing adeptness. During the social events, however, we experienced one of the most enjoyable aspects of crosscultural exchange, that of trying to communicate subtleties and nuances to people who learned English as a second language. (Needless to say, the English speakers were for the most part monolingual and offered very little proficiency speaking Japanese . . . except for *sushi*.) During a conversation at the farewell reception I was asked to explain the phrase, "I came from Alabama, with a banjo on my knee."

The phrase of course was from the American folksong "Oh, Susannah," which was given an impromptu rendition by our Dean, faculty, and student hosts. The confusion seemed to arise from the perceived difficulty of a traveler condemned to journey with "a banjo on my knee." I don't think the explanation attempt did much to clarify the crosslanguage confusion, but at least it provided some good laughs and conviviality at the social event. This reception capped what had been an enriching visit from our Japanese guests. After a stop with lectures at the University of Florida coordinated by Dr. Jay Rosenbek, the group traveled to Florida State University in scenic Tallahassee to enjoy the hospitality and expertise of our students and faculty in the Department of Communication Disorders. We had lectures and demonstrations presented by our faculty on the topics of current research in our NeuroCom-NeuroCog Laboratory; the use of memory books to enhance communication in dementia; objective measurement of lingual function in neuromotor speech disorders and swallowing; and the acoustics and laryngeal pathologies associated with the professional singing voice. Site visits and tours were arranged to Tallahassee Memorial Hospital's Adult Day Services Center, a model respite center for people with dementia and other neurological conditions. The group also visited the Neuroscience Center with its Parkinson Disease and Memory Disorders Specialty Clinics.

The benefits of the visit were certainly reciprocal, and we were able to talk with our Japanese colleagues about care and services in their home country. These were experienced health care professionals who represented nursing, physical therapy, medicine, and speech-language-hearing pathology. It was gratifying to witness the core traits of clinicians emerge during interactions with clients at the Adult Day Services Center. Despite language barriers, these clinicians plunged into helping with the ongoing crafts project (making a handsome string of autumn leaves and beads as decorations for upcoming fall holidays).

A highlight of the visit was the cultural enrichment of social interaction and sharing of regional food. Lunches for our Japanese guests included a pizza and ice cream social ("slices as big as your head" from a local pizzeria) and a regional indoctrination to seafood gumbo and real tidbits of alligator tail prepared with a remoulade sauce. (Surprisingly, the consensus was that the gator tail tasted like chicken.) Real key lime pie (not the green, food-colored goop) topped the regional menu. At each of the social receptions, in Japanese fashion, the group assembled at the end of the evening and sang several Japanese songs for us. These were beautiful musical offerings of autumn, elements of nature, and songs of friendship and camaraderie. The farewell reception, too, was highlighted by delightful Japanese folk songs and dances. We reciprocated with "Oh, Susannah," "I've Been Working on the Railroad," and a rollicking version of "Swing Low, Sweet Chariot." The musical fare concluded with an emotional rendition of "Till We Meet Again" sung by one of our guests Sakura Higashi.

This was the fourth visit to the United States by our Japanese counterparts. I have enjoyed each unique experience. Each is reciprocally rewarding. Each convinces us ever further that parochialism has no role in crosscultural efforts to enhance our skills in dealing with people with communication and cognitive disorders. I hope this issue of our journal with its potpourri of information and clinical research helps our readers learn and improve their practices. Perhaps it will also prompt readers to initiate and nurture exchanges of information and learning that go beyond national borders and extend to the global community of people helping people.

Some things are lost in translation. Some things are gained. This crosscultural visit proved once again that despite the risk of linguistic perplexity, such as wax tadpoles and banjos on the knee, we have much to gain by learning from each other. It's a small world, after all.

CHAPTER 24

SNAKE WINE AND CULTURE SHOCK

Translation between [cultures] is enriching, essential, and impossible.

—Goethe

That extracted paraphrase of Geothe is a little over-the-top but representative of his brilliant irony. Cultural translation and understanding is not impossible, but it is not easy. I write this in the middle of a unique cultural translation in Hong Kong, which is not my home culture. This experience of living in another society has been exhilarating, profoundly rewarding, and at times bewildering. I've done a little reading on the phenomenon of culture shock, and now I know why. Ex-patriots and others who have traveled extensively or lived abroad know culture shock intimately. It is an occupational hazard of being transported in almost Beam-me-up-Scotty fashion into a new environment.

Lalervo Oberg (2002), an anthropologist, has written an insightful piece on cultural shock and adjustment, re-entry shock, and important factors to adjustment. He explains that cultural shock is precipitated by the anxiety that results from losing all of the familiar signs and symbols of your own cultural comfort zone. These signs are the thousands of ways by which we orient ourselves to daily life: when to bow or shake hands when we meet people; when and how to give tips (I recently had experience with this when a tip proffered to a hotel employee who had been very kind was rejected with the comment, "I cannot accept. It's my job."); when to use chopsticks in a communal dish; how to purchase antifungal cream; when and when not to queue up for transportation or services; or how to take photographs without insult or privacy invasion. In a new culture many of these cues are removed or altered. Suddenly one finds oneself not so much like a fish out of water but like a bewildered squid in strange, unfamiliar waters.

Discernable stages of culture shock and cultural adjustment have been identified. Individuals differ greatly in the depth of their experience with culture disharmony, but the symptoms are unmistakable and can be observed in oneself and others. Grousing about inconveniences and embracing your home culture in irrational glorification are two signs. The oft-quoted Ugly American stereotypical question of "How much is that in real money?" is an example of cultural ignorance or insensitivity. Examples abound. "Whenever we're in a foreign country the first thing we seek out is a McDonalds" is another symptom of cultural superficiality. But how far does one go to experience and attempt to learn about another culture? No doubt the answer is buried again among differences across individuals and depth of previous cultural exposure.

Snake wine is a good example. I think it is fair to say that, to many Westerners, the mid winter tonic of snake and noodles or the elixir of a shot of freshly drawn snake blood or snake wine would be a unique experience. My last visit to Hong Kong allowed me to wander the Western districts of Sheung Wan and Sai Ying Pun and discover some of these traditional Chinese venues of serpentine culinary arts. I politely declined an offer of snake wine and later vowed that on my return I would experience some of these cultural variants. So during my three-month residency this time I had another opportunity. While browsing among the wonders of Chinese craft and culture at the Yue Hwa department store, I noticed an impressive display of snake wine at a display table. The woman hawking the nectar offered me a sample from a small paper cup: A huge glass jar of fermenting snakes crowned the display impressively.

These are not benign little garden snakes, but huge, multicolored serpents that would do justice to Eden. I sip-tasted the liquid in genuine oenophile fashion, and then proceeded to toss it down. Lovely. A heady little bouquet with hints of cherry cough medicine, pears, apple, and grass. Probably not being the first Western "tourist" the salesperson had induced to taste her miracle elixir, she then delighted in showing me the ingredients on the wine bottle box, written in English; ". . . snake, tokays, dog, sparrows, . . ." and then some unusual bits and pieces that would best go unmentioned.

Comforted by this foray into cultural encounter, I continued research on some of the medicinal and culinary delights that might be regarded by some as culturally diffuse. The markets and menus are a mother lode of cultural exploration and difference. Dried sea cucumbers; shark fin soup; hundred year old eggs; boiled, boned chicken feet; goose intestines; pig stomach; bird nest soup; sea moss—all these are delicacies that may well test the cultural sensitivity of visitors.

The reward of cultural experience, however, is captured in the small enlightening incidents that not only create the shock but the recompense. One person's shock is another person's recompense. Being a participant observer by joining in activities of the people is a good way to ensure richness of the experience. Factors that are crucial to intercultural adjustment include open mindedness (the ability to keep one's opinions flexible and receptive); communicativeness (ability to inquire and verbalize feelings and thoughts), flexibility (ability to respond or tolerate the ambiguity of new situations); curiosity (the desire to know about other people, places, and ideas); positive expectations (successful intercultural adjustment and positive expectation are highly correlated); tolerance of differences and ambiguities (sympathetic understanding and acceptance of beliefs and practices differing from one's own); and positive regard for others (ability to express warmth, empathy, and respect for others). Oberg (2002) outlines these points as vital factors in adjustment to new cultural environments.

My experience here, through the auspices of my home base at Florida State University and the kindness and support of Paul Fletcher and the faculty, staff, and students at the Department of Speech and Hearing Sciences at the University of Hong Kong, has been culturally and professionally gratifying on several fronts. First, we have had the opportunity to launch collaborative research on the effects of distraction across languages on word retrieval and cognitive performance of bilingual Cantonese-English speakers with aphasia. Second, we have been able to form new professional bonds with several colleagues that will no doubt lead to future reciprocal intercultural exchanges. Third, we have been able to learn from each other and put our sometimes-parochial views and practices into a more global perspective. Fourth, we have been able to enjoy many and bountiful *dim sum* lunches with professional and light-hearted banter as well as the rainbow tastes of tiny shrimp dumplings, sweet sea scallops, honey, walnut, and vegetable won tons, and thinly sliced goose with vinegar garlic sauce. I have learned much from these: not only to tap my fingers twice on the table to thank the tea pourer, but also to nearly always avoid ophthalmic chopstick injury. These are the enrichments of inter-cultural professional familiarity and understanding.

This issue is a veritable *dim sum* of information as well. We offer a series of papers presented at the Academy of Neurological Communication Disorders and Sciences on the ongoing work of the group on the development of practice guidelines. We also have a timely contribution by Sharon Moss on culturally and linguistically sensitive assessment. From Australia we get an important ar-ticle on variability of materials used in dysphagia evaluation. We have a study of script knowledge following stroke. From another center in Australia we have a comprehensive and crucial description of communication disorders in people with HIV. Finally, from a happy valley we have an intriguing contribu-tion on occupational stress in speech-language pathologists working in health-care settings. This issue presents information pertinent to a variety of cultures with in our discipline.

Goethe was not exactly correct. Translation between and among cultures is indeed possible. Nonetheless, he was spot on about the enriching and essen-tial part. Culture shock can be minimized by familiarity and understanding. To that notion I'd raise a small paper cup of snake wine and say "Cheers."

REFERENCE

Oberg, L. (2002). *Culture shock and the problems of adjustment to new cultural environments.* Milwaukee: Worldwide classroom. http://www.worldwide.edu/planning

CHAPTER 25

NEVER ODD OR EVEN

Live not on evil deed; live not on evil.

— A 2002 palindrome

2002. The same forward as backward. A palindrome year. It seems as though I don't remember this happening since 1991. The next one will be 2112. It is quite remarkable that there have not been two palindrome years within a century of each other since 1001. The next two palindromes within a hundred years of each other will be 2992/3003. Maybe we should plan something special.

For those of you in our readership who do not amuse yourselves by inveterate word play, a palindrome is a word, phrase, verse, sentence, or set of numerals that retain the same order in both directions, forward and backward. Many of us who make a living by studying and attempting to figure out language in dissolution are predisposed to revel and, yes, obsess a bit, on the mystique and allure of words. Some of us engage in word play even on the deathbed. An interesting Internet site source of word play and brain candy, *http://www.corsinet.com/braincandy/dying.html,* lists the last words of famous people. The French grammarian, Dominique Bouhours, who died in 1792, is quoted as uttering these last words: "I am about to—or I am going to—die: either expression is correct."

So this palidromiac year is special, and since it follows such a remarkable and tragic 2001 with many in the world expressing uncertainty about the future, perhaps this is a good year to remind ourselves that life continues. One way to do that may well be to pick up the threads of word play and consider how utterly mesmerizing language can be. 2002 is a reminder to do that.

Palindromes are well known to those of us named Bob, Anna, Otto, or Noel Leon. These language quirks are easily spotted in some single-word examples such as *deified, eye, kayak, level, madam, radar, repaper, reviver, rotator,* or *sexes.* Some of the longer constructions, however, begin to toy with the boundaries of obscurity. Classic palindromic quotes have been attributed to the introduction used by an early resident of the Garden of Eden (*Madam, I'm Adam.*), to Napoleon (*Able was I ere I saw Elba.*), and to the civil engineering vision of Theodore Roosevelt (*A man, a plan, a canal—Panama!*). Punctuation never matters in palindromes. Some of these mirrorlike constructions seem almost mystical and profound in their multilevel layers of meaning. We wonder if there is a nuance of meaning that we are missing. Others are less reflective, particularly when traces of incongruity (which, with brevity, truly *is* the co-soul of wit) mushroom into the realm of silly (*I'm a lasagna hog. Go hang a salami.*)

My meta-linguistic research has directed me to those even more preoccupied with palindromic play. People may well have too much time on their hands when they can spend goodly effort on constructing multiple variations on the theme of *A man, a plan, a canal—Panama!* Consider the following:

- A man, a plan, a cat, a canal—Panama!
- A man, a plan, a cat, a ham, a yak, a yam, a hat, a canal—Panama!
- A man, a plan, a canoe, pasta, heros, rajas, a coloratura, maps, snipe, percale, macaroni, a gag, a banana bag, a tan, a tag, a banana bag again, or: a camel, a crepe, pins, spam, a rut, a Rolo, cash, a jar, sore hats, a peon, a canal—Panama!

Palindromes, of course, are not restricted to any one language. From Ernie's Favorite Palindromes (*http://complex.gmu.edu/neural/personnel/ernie/witty/palindromes.html*) we have examples in:

LATIN	*Sum mus.* (I am a mouse.)
	A nap, a lamb, ab mal ap ana. (He who is holy shall not nap with lambs.)
SPANISH	*Anita lava la tina.* (Anita washes the tub.)
PORTUGUESE	*Roma de tem amor.* (Rome has love for me.)
HUNGARIAN	*Mar ujra var a varju ram.* (Once again, the crow is waiting for me.)
FINNISH	*Iso rikas sika sokosakissa kirosi.* (A fat, rich pig cursed in a poker gang.)

So, we contemplate forward-backward linguistic constructions, while Emil, asleep, peels a lime. It is enough to make one want to shout, Yo, Bob, mug a gumbo boy. After a while, these word obsessions get tiring, and we yawn a more Roman way. It is reminiscent of star comedy by democrats. It is almost too hot to hoot. Was it a cat I saw? Dumb mud.

Yes, many of these mirror sentences and phrases are a bit of a stretch. But they are fun, and if nothing else they remind us in this palindromic year of 2002 that the gift of language is truly a marvel. When language is impaired or lost, it is no fun at all. So many of our readers spend each day dealing with people with fractured language, so I guess it is no wonder that we toy with words like a cat with yarn. 2002 is a good year to engage in linguistic recreation.

This issue of our journal is packed with some serious issues involving speech, voice, and language. As you can see by the Table of Contents, we are privileged to have a series of tutorial presentations from a spectrum of experts in human communication and its disorders. Gabbert and colleagues present a tutorial on speech production sequelae associated with psychotropic drugs. Garrett and Deal share with us some clinical techniques and insights on endoscopic and perceptual evaluation of velopharyngeal insufficiency and hypernasality. We have two excellent articles in addition to our tutorials: Dworkin and colleagues report on the use of videoendoscopy for diagnosis and treatment of poor tracheoesophageal speech. From Florida State University, Dijkstra, Bourgeois, Burgio, and Allen offer results of a compelling intervention study on discourse of nursing home residents with dementia and their nursing assistants.

In this issue as well, we are pleased to present a roundtable discussion on approaches to solving the assessment mysteries of disordered voice. Several principal clinical researchers with notable experience on the evaluation of voice disorders present this roundtable forum. We are grateful for their sharing the wealth of their proficiency. One of the participants in this forum was the late Harold A. "Andy" Leeper. Dr. Leeper and his colleagues have been frequent contributors to this journal. His gifts to our profession have been many, and we will miss his insightful research and his warm personality.

So many dynamos. Never odd or even.

CHAPTER 26

THE SOCIOLOGY OF APHASIA

'Twixt the optimist and pessimist
The difference is droll:
The optimist sees the doughnut
But the pessimist sees the hole.

—McLandburgh Wilson, *Optimist and Pessimist* (Augarde, 1991)

Half empty? Half full? Doughnut? Hole? Perspective is a marvelous leveler. These days the concept of dispositional optimism is getting a great deal of play in the behavioral science literature as well as in the popular press. In a world tipped asunder with occult terrorism, territorial and religious conflict, zealotry, and improbability, the collective psyche has undergone some unprecedented transformation. It seems easy to become disenchanted. A few short kilometers away are the dreadful provinces of pessimism and cynicism. In my casual observations of personality trait evolution, there seems to be a fairly clear-cut developmental progression. A person who develops the perceptual bias of filtering only the negative is a pessimist in training. And a good pessimist is well on the road to becoming a cynic, a person who can find nothing good or favorable anywhere. One of the dictionary definitions of a cynic is one who is bitterly or sneeringly distrustful, contemptuous, or pessimistic. Cynicism has an even more lurid etymology if one looks at the Greek origins of the word. One meaning of the term *kynikós* is "doglike, currish. . .resembling the actions of a snarling dog" (*Random House Unabridged Dictionary*, 2nd ed., 1987). Not exactly the ideal roommate.

External events that reek with adversity have a way of forcing people to re-examine what it means to be well, happy, or positive. These events can be societal and even global, such as the wretched events following September 11, 2001; or they can be deeply internal and personal, such as the aftermath of neural explosions in the head. Stroke and resulting aphasia have an increasingly recognized impact on the psychosocial well-being of persons who experience it. Yet, remarkably, relatively little empirical research attention has been directed toward these issues of disability. We see a little more attention given to social models of aphasia, but much of the research effort appears to be directed still to the neurology and neurolinguistics of the disorder. These efforts are vital and have given us a superb grounding in the holy grail quest for an adequate theory of aphasia. Much needed, however, is theoretical integration of some of the psychosocial ramifications of the disability. I have argued this issue in a recent publication entitled *The science of aphasia: From theory to therapy* (LaPointe, 2002). Social models of aphasia are gaining acceptance, and I would go so far as to suggest that we need to define and clarify a research direction and agenda that might best be captured by the rubric "the sociology of aphasia."

SOCIAL MODELS OF APHASIA

Models of aphasia that incorporate social elements as vital signs of a living, growing scientific and clinical discipline are increasingly apparent. The medical model of the assessment, diagnosis, and treatment of the acute phase of aphasia is no longer as appropriate as translated earlier. Certainly, aphasia is associated with certain unalienable medical conditions and constructs; and these should neither be ignored nor abandoned. But aphasia is also social. It is based on communicating, interacting with others, and living in a societal context.

The isolation and imposed withdrawal seen in so many people with aphasia may well be iatrogenic, or caused by the intervention. The relevance of knee-to-knee individual sessions of drill on word retrieval and phonologic precision ("Name the picture. Point to your head. Point to your feet. Say no *ifs, ands, or buts.*") may well be approaching passé for all but a few process-oriented conditions. In Scandinavia, Australia, South Africa, Canada, the United Kingdom, Japan, and other parts of the globe, international conferences on treatment approaches for aphasia are increasingly imbued with elements of social context and interaction needs of communicators (LaPointe, 2002).

A confluence of elements has begun to shape the flow of aphasia treatment. Fitting well into social models of aphasia is the recently articulated Life Participation Approach to Aphasia. The American Speech-Language-Hearing Association (ASHA) sponsored and encouraged a group of clinical aphasiologists and scholars in what has become known as the Life Participation Approach to Aphasia Project (LPAA) Project Group (2001).

An area of deep mystery within the area of the sociology of aphasia is the business of adaptation, accommodation, and adjustment to chronicity. Not all aphasia goes away. Few people with the disability are returned to premorbid baselines of function or of life participation. We have paid too little attention to these cutting issues. Holland (2001) has commented on reasons for optimism about aphasia rehabilitation and particularly about rehabilitative efforts that highlight living with aphasia. She presented an invited lecture at the sesquicentennial of our university on topics such as the rise of group intervention as a viable modality of intervention, and support. She highlighted as well the benefits inherent in shifting the focus of aphasia treatment from impairments to the new ICIDH-2 Beta 2 models that emphasize outcomes related to activity and participation. With the rise of group modes of intervention, it becomes quite typical to hear participants with aphasia reiterate the issues of chronicity and adaptation that are echoes of all who have faced these storms. When the wreck of aphasia occurs, the big questions surface and recur. How does one accept a radically tilted life? How does a family adjust to a life that may be tenfold the challenge on Friday what it was on Monday? Is it possible to deal with chronicity and a prodigiously changed existence? Can relative happiness ever be attained or regained? Is there precedent for dealing with the illness experience? How does one cope with chronicity? How does one live with aphasia? We need a research agenda on coping with chronicity and specifically on coping with aphasia. Some recent research on general aspects of successful aging and coping speaks to both the issue of adaptation to chronicity as well as attitudes of dispositional optimism.

KEYS TO SUCCESSFUL AGING AND COPING

In the United States longitudinal research conducted at Harvard University has revealed interesting lifestyle attributes or keys that are alleged to be associated with successful aging, wellness, and positive life quality. George E. Vaillant and his associates have conducted longitudinal studies over a duration of more than 30 years (Vaillant & Mukamal, 2001). Vaillant and several of his colleagues through the years followed three demographic groups (*n* = 824). One cohort was comprised of Harvard University graduates, one of inner city Boston men, and one of gifted California women. These groups were given psychological and medical tests, physical examinations, and interviews by psychiatrists. They were asked to evaluate their lives and feelings. Some of these groups were followed and evaluated for up to 40 years. The evaluations and perceptions of a large group between the ages of 60 and 80 years were analyzed and three distinct groups emerged: a group characterized as the "happy well;" one labeled the "sad sick" (who had various ailments and decreased perception of enjoyment of life); and a group called the "prematurely dead" (a subset of participants who had died prior to the age of 60). The study is fraught with complexity and defies oversimplification, but some of the conclusions rendered by Vaillant and his associates are difficult to ignore. The personal attributes that characterized the happy well group (and qualities that were remarkably less prevalent in the other two groups) included:

- Orientation toward the future—the ability to anticipate, plan, and hope
- Gratitude, forgiveness, and optimism—the classic views of important life lessons during adversity and generally perceiving bottles, cups, and glasses and life events as half full rather than half empty
- Empathy—the ability to imagine the world as it seems to the other person (this is strikingly close to the concept of "theory of mind," which has attracted considerable research interest in people with right hemisphere damage.)
- Reaching out—the desire to do things *with* other people, not to do things *to* them; or the rumination that other people keep doing things *to* us

The Harvard studies also pointed out the positive aspects of support systems and of participation in societal and community activities. It is not difficult to see the links among all of these concepts that have been associated with positive and successful aging and coping to the chronicity of aphasia. Surely the functional, pragmatic, and life participation approaches reviewed and advocated here are vehicles for facilitating successful life with aphasia (LaPointe, 2000; 2002).

Gigantic questions remain. How do we identify societal, community, and family system traits that nurture coping? How can we nurture or facilitate successful coping? What life participation outcomes reveal successful intervention? What nature or nurture elements are responsible for the development and maintenance of positivism? How do we avoid the snarling dogs in the briar patch of cynicism? How can we get people to view the doughnut and not just the hole? Perhaps we shall make progress on the answer to these questions as we more clearly define a research agenda on the sociology of aphasia.

And so we present another issue of our journal, which is jam-packed with ideas and articles designed to help you cope with your daily challenges, be they from external or internal forces. Try to see the doughnut, not just the hole.

REFERENCES

Augarde, T. (1991). *The Oxford dictionary of modern quotations.* New York: Oxford University Press.

Holland, A. L. (2001). *The pony in the bedroom: Optimism about aphasia rehabilitation.* Sesquicentennial Lecture presented at Florida State University.

LaPointe, L. L. (2000). Quality of life with brain damage. *Brain and Language, 71,* 135–137.

LaPointe, L. L. (2002). Functional and pragmatic directions in aphasia treatment. *The sciences of aphasia (Volume. 1): From theory to therapy.* In R. de Bleser & I. Papathanasiou (Eds.) Oxford: Elsevier Science Ltd.

LPAA Project Group (2001). *Life participation approach to aphasia: A statement of values for the future. http://www.asha.org/speech/disabilitions/LPAA.cfm*

Vaillant, G. E. & Mukamal, K. (2001). Successful aging. *American Journal Psychiatrics, 158* (June), 839.

CHAPTER 27

PROVERBS

Proverbs are short sentences drawn from long experience.

—Cervantes, *Don Quixote* (1814)

O ne good thing about being wrong is the joy it brings to others.

Your problem is never your problem.

Your reaction to your problem is your problem.

Some people drink deeply from the fountain of knowledge while others merely gargle.

Your manuscript is both good and original; but the part that is good is not original, and the part that is original is not good.

Next to the originator of a good sentence is the first quoter of it.

The early bird gets the worm.

None of the previous sentences is original. (Is anything?) This is a string of old-fangled and new-fangled proverbs and sayings. The World Wide Web is full of sites with information about proverbs and lists of pithy sayings that are categorized in all kinds of ways. One of the best schemes is to view these gems of wisdom (or obviousness) chronologically. One can observe either plagiarism in action or the historical redundancy of good ideas. Another scheme is to view proverbs by alleged country of origin, although here as well one can see the same kernels of wisdom cropping up across continent and culture.

As many of the sites that provide lists of sayings attest, proverbs are thought to contain the essence of wisdom. Real nuggets. The quintessence of wise. Wisdom comes from experience, and of course, experience comes from making mistakes. So, proverbs are largely a record of the world's mistakes, distilled into a single phrase, and turned into an example for people who follow. These terse life lessons have been passed on across and within generations and cultures, many times by oral tradition. Even today, each of us has a personal collection of these lessons that have been drilled into us largely by teachers and parents designed to give us a plan or a clue and largely through oral redundancy. Some even have been categorized as "Momisms," those oft-repeated supposed truisms designed to create perfect offspring. "Waste not; want not" was one of the mealtime favorites in my youth, perpetrated by depression-era parents for whom waste was equated with sin. Some lessons work too well.

A recently published book on the subject is a delightful and informative work by Linda and Roger Flavell (1997) entitled *Dictionary of Proverbs and Their Origins*. This tome contains over 400 proverbs and has traced the origins of hundreds of them, listing their general meaning, variations on the theme, and a history of usage.

The origins of some are indeed interesting even if quite predictable. For example, "Speak of the devil" or its variant theme "Talk of the devil and he will appear" apparently comes from the ancient fable in which a wolf appears whenever it is mentioned. The proverb "An elephant never forgets" comes by way of another animal for there is an ancient Greek saying that "Camels never forget an injury." Apparently, the camel's capacity for memory has been generalized to the long-living elephant as well. "Look before you leap" is rooted in Aesop's fable *The Fox and the Goat* from 570 BC.

It doesn't take much of a perusal of proverbs to discover that contradictions are rife among the listings. One web site (www.shoal.net.au/~seabreeze/proverbs .html) sets up this approach-avoidance situation by the following arrangements of contradictory advice:

Look before you leap. . .*but*. . .He who hesitates is lost.

Many hands make light work. . .*but*. . .Too many cooks spoil the broth.

Silence is golden. . .*but*. . .The squeaky wheel gets the grease.

If you lie down with dogs you'll get up with fleas. . .*but*. . .If you can't beat 'em, join 'em.

Contemporary proverbs are also rampant and multiplying like lagomorphs. Many of these are infused with references to technology. A few examples are

A journey of a thousand sites begins with a single click.

Fax is stranger than fiction.

Home is where your @ is.

The geek shall inherit the earth.

Speak softly and carry a cellular phone.

That last bit of advice is becoming ever more prescient as social distain and verbal conflict increase between boorish users of mobile phones and those of us in restaurants, classrooms, and even houses of worship, who have no interest in hearing about the magnificent importance of the latest business deal or what time the babysitter will arrive.

This issue of our journal has another pastiche of important offerings. We have an article by Sapir and colleagues that characterizes the voice and speech abnormalities of Parkinson disease with a variety of demographic and medical variables. Coelho and Pobb present an acoustic analysis with proposed explanatory models of that relatively rare condition known as foreign accent syndrome. We also have a clinical note on multidisciplinary assessment of visual spatial neglect in a bilingual patient, and a technical note on voltage and light source influences on photoglottography. Also in this issue is the first of what will be a series of articles emanating from committees coordinated by the Academy of Neurologic Communication Disorders and Sciences on practice guidelines for neurogenic communication and cognitive disorders. This first article, as explained by Golper in the ANCDS Bulletin Board, focuses on the disorder of dysarthria. Other practice guidelines will follow, and these should prove to be invaluable references for researchers and practitioners who deal with people with neurologically-based disorders.

Perhaps the wisdom contained in this issue will give rise to some proverbs of tomorrow. I leave you with good wishes for a happy and productive holiday season as well as a final proverbial contradiction:

On the one hand. . .
Hold fast the words of your ancestors.

But beware that. . .
Wise men make proverbs and fools repeat them.

REFERENCES

Cervantes Saavedra, M. (1814). *Don Quixote.* New York: David Huntington.

Flavell, L., & Flavell, R. (1997). *Dictionary of proverbs and their origins.* New York: Barnes & Noble, Inc.

CHAPTER 28

LAUGH PILLS

The beauty of the world has two edges, one of laughter, one of anguish, cutting the heart asunder.

—Virginia Woolf, *A Room of One's Own* (1929)

Sometimes laughter and anguish are pretty difficult to discern. They can be so interwoven that their colors blend. Virginia Woolf recognized the strange relationship between anguish and laughter. One can precede the other. One can cause the other. Both, in fact, may be necessary ingredients of the beauty of the world. As the cliché suggests, it is difficult to appreciate the finer points of honey without an experience of vinegar. So, too, with some of our baser human emotions. Some of the very best humorists in the world of literature have arisen from tormented backgrounds. Humor has a well-documented association with wellness; to view it as one of the most potent coping mechanisms available to primates is not a stretch.

That jokes and humor can arise from the ashes of suffering and anguish was no more apparent to me than at a recent meeting of the California Speech-Language-Hearing Association (CSHA) convention in Monterey, California. Against the magnificent backdrop of the Central California Coast, professionals in speech-language-hearing pathology from Del Norte to Point Loma gathered to continue their professional education across a comprehensive range of topics. They were also in for a surprise or two. At least *I* was.

The headliner at the association banquet was a speaker/entertainer named Kathy Buckley who bills herself as "America's first hearing-impaired comedienne." Ms. Buckley had an astonishing routine and a remarkable story to tell. (Much of it is available on her website, *http://www.kathybuckley.com*) Kathy Buckley has an impressive resumé of performances with appearances on quite a few high-profile American comedy shows, including guest appearances or profiles on *The Tonight Show, The Today Show, Good Morning America, CBS This Morning, Entertainment Tonight*, and dozens of others. Ms. Buckley was also the subject of *I Can Hear the Laughter*, a 1991 Emmy award-winning documentary. Though by most standards she has received a good deal of national exposure, her story is still not as well known or recognized as it should be. Kathy Buckley is a very funny person. Her humor arises from her life experiences, many of which have been horrendous; but she has wrapped these experiences in life lessons that personify the spirit of battlers everywhere who have fought back from adversity and even drawn from it and laughed about it. It becomes quickly apparent that Kathy Buckley's humor has another purpose. She says that she loves to make people laugh, but she loves it even more if she can teach them something at the same time.

Kathy was raised in Ohio, and her hearing loss was not detected until she was in the second grade. She tells a tale of early years characterized by misdiagnosis and mishandling. "I was in a school for the retarded for two years before they found out I was hearing impaired," she says. "And they call *me* slow. . ."

After high school, she narrates, "I went through one hell after another." She suffered internal injuries from an automobile accident and required 32 stitches in her face. At age 20, she was run over by a 3,500 pound lifeguard Jeep while sunbathing on a beach. From this she suffered intermittent paralysis in her lower limbs and was treated for five years for the residuals of the day at the beach. A year later, she was diagnosed with cervical cancer and went through two more years of hospitalization and treatment.

Despite this saga, which could well sink even the strongest, Kathy turned these tragedies into springboards of opportunity. She began to collect national attention in about 1992 when she was selected from among hundreds of performers to tell her story at the National Association for Campus Activities Convention. From there she became a favorite on the college campus circuit, and her recognition continues to grow.

At the CSAH Convention in Monterey, Kathy had an audience of experts in communication disorders howling with laughter at her jokes and clever observational humor. She also had them weeping at the poignancy of her advocacy born of her personal story. Kathy Buckley demonstrates once again that from the ashes of anguish, humor is born; that the emotion of mirth can displace depression; and that laughter truly is an exceptional pill. If you get a chance, do not miss the opportunity to hear this remarkable woman.

This issue of our journal presents a broad palette of offerings as well, extending from mouse larynx to glossectomy. From Queensland comes an article that is the result of the fusion of interests of geneticists and speech/voice scientists. This research suggests that the unique functional characteristics of the intrinsic laryngeal muscles may be based in laryngeal muscle-specific gene expression. This may set the table for future laryngeal muscle-specific genetic research on the development of new treatments for laryngeal muscle dysfunction. Once again, we see that the bridge between basic research and application is not so ethereal. Following this research is a study that provides physiologic evidence and explanation of the effects of a frequently used voice therapy technique, that of manual circumlaryngeal manipulation. In another contribution from international scientists, Tara Whitehill and colleagues from the University of Hong Kong describe speech errors associated with dental abnormalities in Cantonese speakers. The issue concludes with two case studies: one of recovery of communication skills following intracerebral hemorrhage and another from India on the use of a tongue prosthesis for a patient with total glossectomy.

Virginia Woolf may have underestimated the dichotomous nature of the world. The beauty of the world has at least two edges. This issue of the journal explores several and may well contribute to a new facet or two. While reading and learning from the tragedies of others, remember the medicinal value of laugh pills. They prevent the heart from being cut asunder.

REFERENCE

Woolf, V. (1929). *A room of one's own.* New York: Harcourt, Brace.

CHAPTER **29**

SAGE ADVICE

...science is like a beautiful cloud of gold and scarlet that diffuses wondrous hues of beams of light in the west. It is not an illusion, but the splendor and beauty of truth. However, now the cloud rises, the winds blow it over the fields, and it takes on darker, more somber colors. It is performing a task and changing its party clothes—think of it as putting on its work shirt. (p. 26)

—Santiago Ramóny Cajal (1897)

B rown bag discussions in academia can be most fruitful. Not only can colleagues grapple with ideas but with tuna on rye. A few weeks ago I was invited to share a brown bag lunch with our cluster of doctoral students at Florida State University. They gather regularly and wrestle with theoretic and practical academic challenges against the crunch-slurp backdrop of celery and lowfat yogurt. This time they invited me to join them and wear my toque of editor so we could discuss such issues as "How do we get published?" "What are editors looking for?" "How do we get started?" and, "How do we transform the process of scientific writing to be less like being dragged behind a slow-moving train?"

Both our conclusions and our brown bags were healthful and scanty. We debated and discussed the fairness of the perception of tier one, tier two, and tier n journals in our discipline; the criteria used to evaluate the relative merit of publication in various outlets; and criteria that some use to determine if published works are "trash or treasures." No easy issues these. We pondered the peer review process and the unsettling trend for some students to depend too heavily on nonpeer reviewed sources accessed via the Internet. Not far into the discussion I was able to recommend several of the sources that came to mind on the general topic of advice to young scientists. One that is particularly informative, if somewhat brushed with the bias of the location and time it was written, is Ramón y Cajal's *Advice for a young investigator* (2000). This latest edition is another version of his sage advice first disseminated in 1897 and subsequently in several later variations. As the translators N. and L. W. Swanson indicate, Santiago Ramón y Cajal was a mythic figure in science. Many contemporary neuroscientists regard him as one of the fathers of modern neurobiology. He did years of laborious research on histology and methods of staining neural specimens that culminated in a published work that reassessed the structure of the nervous system. His legacy was variegated. He slaved in the laboratory doing cellular level research. But he always revered the role of mentor and accepted the challenge of attempting to teach and comfort young scientists.

Refreshingly, he also had a rich sense of humor that comes through in his writings, especially when he skewers eccentric scientists by amplifying their stereotypic images. For example, as he attempts to advise young scientists, he warns them not to become the "types" he has encountered. One such type is the "contemplator." In the words of Ramón y Cajal, "We have all seen teachers who are wonderfully talented and full of energy and initiative—with ample facilities at their disposal—who never produce any original work and almost never write anything" (p. 76).

Another interesting species is the "instrument addict." Ramón y Cajal blasts broadside.

This rather unimportant variety of ineffectualist can be recognized immediately by a sort of fetishistic worship of research instruments. They are as fascinated by a gleam of metal as the lark is with its own reflection in a mirror. They lovingly care for the objects of their idolatry, which are kept as polished as mirrors and a beautifully displayed as images in a cathedral. (p. 81)

Although his book of advice to young scientists is replete with the necessity for binding good hypotheses to theories, and the reward of advancing or developing a theory, he also does an adequate job of satirizing the "professional" theorist.

These are highly cultivated, wonderfully endowed minds whose wills suffer from a particular form of lethargy, which is all the more serious because it is not apparent to them and is usually not thought of as being particularly important. . . . They claim to view things on a grand scale; they live in the clouds. (p. 84)

These are examples that show the wit and rapier of this renowned scientist. But throughout the book there is much more than satire. Ramón y Cajal gives timeless advice on beginner's traps, intellectual qualities, what newcomers should know, and social factors beneficial to scientific work. On social factors, he was a product of his times, and although he presents some provocative and archaic ideas on what the scientist should look for in a mate, in my view he is way out of step with his advice: "Ideas are blossoms of virtue that fail to open their petals and wilt quickly in the fumes of boisterous partying" (p. 101). Obviously, this staunch scientist needed to mix up a few bowls of his native Spanish sangria and flamenco about the lab a bit.

This Spanish legend also advises moderation in rebutting attack from other schools or camps. He suggests that getting embroiled in issues of historical precedence and spending too much time on embittering quarrels and debate should be avoided. Although he recognizes the place of legitimate scientific debate, he suggests that some people make a living of it, and never get on with any real discovery because of preoccupation with the chesslike gamesmanship of argument to the point of self-stimulation. Santiago Ramón y Cajal puts it delicately. "When unjustly attacked and forced to defend ourselves, let us do so nobly. Unsheathe your sword, but with tip blunted—adorned with a bouquet of flowers" (p. 129).

Advice to young scientists. Advice to beginning professionals. What a cherished role we have when our advice is solicited. Let us do so wisely, as Ramón y Cajal suggested. We don't want to aspirate our tuna.

This issue of our journal has a variety of exceptional offerings. We have as well two timely articles presented through the collaboration we have established with the Academy of Neurologic Communication Disorders and Sciences. These are solicited articles on *Brain plasticity and recovery from hemiplegia* by Mark Hallett, M.D., from the National Institute of Neurological Disorders and Stroke in Bethesda, Maryland, and *Neurophysiologic basis of rehabilitation* by Leslie Gonzalez Rothi from the Brain Rehabilitation Research Center in Gainesville, Florida. Each of these contributions marks a new and exciting era in brain recovery research. The accumulating confluence of evidence on neurophysiologic change and reorganization that accompany and *are the result of* intervention efforts is indeed a heartening epoch to those of us dedicated to neurologic rehabilitation. We offer as well the results of a study on the preparation of speech-language pathologists on dealing with tracheoesophageal puncture and another on the effects of intensive phonatory-respiratory treatment on voice in two individuals with multiple sclerosis. We also include a book review in this issue on supervision strategies. So don your work shirt, roll up your sleeves, and prepare to examine the beautiful cloud of both science and practice.

REFERENCE

Ramón y Cajal, S. (2000). *Advice for a young investigator*. (N. Swanson & L. W. Swanson, Trans.). Cambridge, MA: The MIT Press.

CHAPTER 30

HOLIDAYS AND YOUTH

*Youth is given. One must put it away like a doll in a closet,
take it out and play with it only on holidays.*

—May Swenson, *How To Be Old* (1963)

What a depressing thought. We can only express our youth on holidays? Is youth to be put away like a doll in a closet and taken out only on holidays? I hope not. I am sure May Swenson was speaking *lingua en bucca* as she composed her sardonic commentary on how to be old.

To the way of thinking of many experts in gerontology, the process of aging is as much attitude as it is biology. We all know examples of 80 year olds who hike Superstition Wilderness trails and are fit, enriched, and open to all that life has to offer. They contradict the stereotypes of aging that we have been inundated with by thousands of messages a day. Wag and Jumbo are good examples. They are the nicknamed and delightful Australian parents of one of our friends from Queensland who, though they are in their seventh decade roaring up to the eighth, live active and enriched lives. Jumbo, the five-foot-tall mother of our friend, bushwalks (hikes) with the best of them; and we remember well the day when she raced up a trail and river bank without even breathing hard, only to stick a foot on the lower strand of barbed wire and raise the upper strand to allow us to catch our breath and plod through the opening. Many 40 year olds could not do as well, do not look as fit, and do not laugh or enjoy life nearly as much.

Perhaps a sense of holiday helps. Aging, youth, wellness, and holiday are strangely connected concepts that are being studied rigorously by those interested in the Fountain of Holiday. As this is being written, with the November and December holidays looming ever nearer, we are reminded of the relationship between holiday and youth by May Swenson and the idea that youth is not just for special occasions.

This issue is in the hands of our readers in March 2001; and, in some lands, March is a month not brimming over with traditionally prominent holidays. However, the calendar reveals there are ample opportunities for joyousness and the celebration of youth on such fine occasions as St. Patrick's Day in the United States and Ireland. In the states, this calls for green beer, corned beef and cabbage, and carefully overboiled potatoes to help celebrate the mythical expungement of serpents from Ireland. It is indeed a jovial, nearly universally celebrated holiday when Lithuanian, Icelandic, and Apache can masquerade as Irish, dress in green, and embrace a festive mood. Aside from Mardi Gras or Carnival in southern climes, two classic golden chances to drop the mundane and engage in prolonged and partially clad revelry, there are few holiday opportunities in March. Of course, there is Mothering Sunday in the United Kingdom and Canberra Day in Australia, but these commemoratives seem ill-suited to reckless abandonment and picking up the threads of our childhood.

So, in search of further March opportunities for extracting our youth from storage, we offer a few celebratory occasions perhaps not usually acknowledged. Only a cursory cruise through several Internet sites reveals a plethora of prospects for merriment. For example, at least in the United States, March is Foot Health Month, National Furniture Refinishing Month, National Frozen Food Month, and National Noodle Month. More specific chances for revelry include March 1 as National Pig Day and March 2 as Old Stuff Day. For the researchers among our readership, March 4 is Holy Experiment Day, and for those who are required to engage in teaching, research, and service, March 5 is Multiple Personalities Day. March 11 marks two reasons for celebration in that it is both Johnny Appleseed Day and Worship of Tools Day. Further feast can be accomplished on March 24, which is National Chocolate Covered Raisins Day (National Chocolate Covered Sultanas Day in Australia). A couple of other interesting entries include March 27 as National "Joe" Day. Further research on this day reveals that everyone who hates his or her name has a right on this day to have everyone they know address them as Joe. Finally, the month of uncanny holidays is rounded out on March 28 by Something on a Stick Day and on March 31 by National Clams on the Half Shell Day.

These unusual March holidays are courtesy of a website devoted to Bizarre March Holidays (*http://library.thinkquest.org/2886/mar.htm*). They are good reminders of a few more serious points. Youth, or a sense of life enjoyment, is not just to be dusted off on holidays; and every day can be a holiday if we are passionate about our work. Work does not have to be slogging drudgery. Fun and work are not incompatible. Aging is not devoid of carnival. Or, maybe another paradoxical way of viewing it is that aging is not devoid of youth. The stereotypes of agism are among the last bastions of general awareness of the danger of "*isms*," be they racism, sexism, or any of the other evil "*isms*" that prey on stereotype and taint the human spirit.

In this issue, we present excellent research from professionals in the serious business of dealing with the daily tragedies of loss of communication, some of whom I know do not regard their work as total drudgery. The process is labored, but the outcome of these many efforts is indeed worthy of holiday. These endeavors may instruct us, inspire us, and in some instances actually improve the practice of what we do. That is good reason to celebrate. This issue includes diverse accomplishments. We have a fine review paper on specific language impairment that addresses thorny issues of definition, causal mechanisms, and neurobiological factors. We also have research by Ross and Wertz that addresses type and severity of aphasia with an eye on life impact during the first seven months poststroke. Other contributions include study of attentional demands and speech timing in Parkinson Disease; normative values on word fluency measures; communication interaction differences among natural speakers and users of augmentative-alternative communication; and a series of eight case studies on assessment and management of dysphagia following pharyngolaryngectomy with free jejunal interposition.

These contributions will instruct us and enlighten us. May we also be reminded that the spirit of youth and festivity are not to be reserved for special occasions, and that just about anything can serve as a good excuse for holiday.

REFERENCES

Anonymous. (2000). *http://library.thinkquest.org/2886/mar.htm*

Swenson, M. (1963). *How to be old.* New York: Scribner.

CHAPTER 31

St. Anthony and Motor Speech

While treasures lost are found again. When young or old thine aid implore.

—Julian of Spires (1231)

S an Antonio, Texas, the river city in the Southwestern United States, was founded by a band of Spanish explorers and missionaries in 1691. Because it was the feast day of St. Anthony, they named the river "San Antonio." Eventually, in 1772 immigrants from a group of islands in the Atlantic established a settlement. Prior to that, of course, the area along the river had been inhabited for centuries by Native Americans, who called the area "Yangaguana," which means "refreshing waters."

In early February of the year 2000, another band of explorers visited San Antonio and met for several days at the biennial conference on Motor Speech and Motor Speech Disorders to present, discuss, debate, and generate ideas on research. The focus of interest was on trying to understand and explain the complex and intricate movements that relate to human speech production and to explore ways of finding or restoring these speech treasures when they become lost.

Curiously, and somewhat tangentially, the researchers and clinicians who gathered in San Antonio in February of 2000 had a few things in common with the namesake of the city of San Antonio. Nearly everywhere, some believers exist who feel that St. Anthony is an efficient intercessor to facilitate help in the return of things lost or stolen. Many believers turn almost reflexively to St. Anthony to help them find lost keys, checkbooks, underwear, and even loves. Those who feel perhaps too familiar with St. Anthony may implore, "Tony, Tony, turn around. Something's lost and must be found."

The reason for invoking St. Anthony's help in finding lost or stolen things is traced to an incident in his own life. St. Anthony of Padua was a teacher and scholar who lost an important book that was allegedly taken by a novice who had grown tired of religious life and decided to leave the community. Anthony implored that the book be returned to him, and legend has it that the thieving novice returned the book of psalms and returned to the Order, forgiven. Since then, the legend has become embellished and has engendered widespread belief that St. Anthony is the one to whom to pray or wish for the return of lost items.

The Internet has some curious sources of information, as we continue to discover in this technologically drenched new century. In researching this connection between San Antonio and searchers for lost treasures, I also learned that especially in Portugal, Italy, France, and Spain, St. Anthony is the patron saint of sailors, travelers, and fisherpersons as well. According to some sources, his statue is sometimes placed in a shrine on the ship's mast, and sailors may scold the saint if he doesn't respond quickly enough to their requests. In addition to these aspects of his job description, St. Anthony also is regarded by some as a holy matchmaker and a guide for charitable givers. St. Anthony's Bread has become a term associated with charitable donations of food to the poor in return for favors granted. This legend has its origin from at least two sources. One holds that a child drowned near the Basilica of St. Anthony that was being built, and the child's mother promised that if the child was restored to her she would give to the poor an amount of corn equal to the child's weight. Her prayer and promise were allegedly rewarded with the boy's return to breath and life. No mention is made of cardiopulmonary resuscitation. A second legend holds that a baker in France was faced with a broken lock on her shop door. She prayed to St. Anthony that the door could be opened by the locksmith without breaking it down and promised bread for the poor in return for the favor. The door was opened, her promise kept, and since then, gifts of food for the poor in response to a favor granted has been referred to as St. Anthony's Bread.

So the connection between St. Anthony, San Antonio, and Motor Speech does have a strange interlacing. When the treasure of speech is lost, we need all the help we can get in attempting to restore it. Another avenue in this quest for things lost is science. So San Antonio was an appropriate setting for the pursuit and dissemination of the latest neuroscientific and clinical information on understanding and restoring lost speech.

This issue is our second that is totally devoted to the proceedings of this Conference on Motor Speech. Monica McHenry, Ph.D., has served as the very capable Special Editor of these papers, and we are proud to publish them within the same year that the conference was held. As you can see from the table of contents, the topics range from speech motor learning and neurophysiological monitoring of the orofacial system in infants to case studies of individuals with dysarthrias from a range of neuropathological conditions. We think this issue of our journal contains a particularly broad and valuable archive of the latest research on speech motor control and neuromotor speech disorders, and we look forward to a continuing collaboration with the conference.

Speech is a fortune. When it is lost, the contemporary scientists who have devoted their professional careers to understanding it and restoring it are indeed following in the footsteps of other legendary finders of lost treasures.

REFERENCES

History of San Antonio: Cited on http://sanantoniocvb.com/history.html

Julian of Spires. Cited on American Catholic Education Internet site: http://listserv.american.edu/catholic/franciscan/anthony/devotion.html

CHAPTER 32

SAGUAROS AND DOGWOODS: CHANGE AND ETHICS

Most of the change we think we see in life is due to truths being in and out of favor.

—Robert Frost, *North of Boston* (1914)

The ever-whirling wheel of change can sometimes make us dizzy. Sometimes it is planned and expected and evolves us. Sometimes it is abrupt and startles us. Change affects each of the concentric circles of our existence. Global, societal, cultural, and familial changes mark us as individuals. Are we ever the same? Are we never constant? Can we poke our finger in the water of the same river twice? Change and constancy are seemingly incongruous states, but we know better. As oxymoronic as the constancy of change appears, we understand it. It is as easy to understand as the seeming contradictory riddle of why a blackberry is red when it is green. Professions change. Practices change. Families and children change. Pictures and videos stop time in its tracks, and still it startles us when we review these and note changes in age and appearance. We are surprised at how our grandparents looked when they were young. We are carried along in the stream of change and soon the milestones of our children's intellectual and physical transformations are blended and fused into the present.

I was particularly reminded of the impact of familial change recently during a meeting of three of my university colleagues on our departmental Personnel and Budget Committee. We broke from the laborious and sometimes odious task of calculating and ranking the performance of our peers to distribute the few crumbs of merit salary increase and chatted about families for a few seconds. One junior faculty member commented on her 3 hours of sleep the night before as she attended and comforted a baby and a toddler with earaches. Another colleague commented on his teenager's spurt of intellectual-spiritual growth when she announced at dinner the night before that she had decided not to attend church with the family and instead would like to invite them to consider conversion to Buddhism with her. The third faculty member revealed the grief and pain in his family by the simultaneous divorce of a daughter and the breakup of a son's long-time love relationship. It seemed as though the marionette children were coming off their strings and wandering randomly into the audience. And so it goes. Three close-to-home cross-sectional examples of the constancy of change and responsibility. The river flows on and we pause and reflect on change and constancy only rarely during milestones such as birthdays, graduations, weddings, and job changes.

For eons, philosophers have speculated on the effect of change on individuals, families, cultures, and societies. How do members of societies cope with the mishmash of evolving influences on one another? What prevents chaos? How is anarchy avoided, if it is avoided? Part of the answer must be rooted (no Australian pun intended) in the emergence of codes of conduct and philosophies of the ancient Greek thinkers. Aristotle, Plato, Socrates, Hippocrates, and Diabetes all struggled with the formation of codification of laws and principles of behavior that would allow cultures to avert chaos and randomness of behavior. Professions have struggled with this as well in the centuries since the Golden Age of Greece.

The treatises on Ethics of the early thinkers have influenced organizations and professions and spawned codes of ethics or codes of conduct that govern and direct. The American Speech-Language-Hearing Association (ASHA), for example, has a defined and regularly revised Code of Ethics that sets forth the fundamental principles and rules considered essential to preserve the highest standards of integrity as the members of the professions discharge their obligations. ASHA's Board of Ethics also maintains a vigorous and active interest in educating its members and the public about issues of ethics that are relevant to our professions. On the ASHA website (www.asha.org), postings of interest include the organization's Code of Ethics and a variety of Board of Ethics statements. In addition 16 detailed statements are contained in a section entitled "Issues in Ethics." These statements are wide ranging and cover topics from Conflicts of Professional Interest to Public Announcements and Public Statements.

The ASHA website also has a statement about change and the effects of the dynamism of the 1990s on our professions. This posted Statement, Responding to the Changing Needs of Speech-Language Pathology and Audiology Students, is a succinct and useful update for practitioners, academics and students. A Professional Issues Bulletin Board also is a forum for individual questions, postings, and interactions among visitors to the website. ASHA's published and posted Ethics Roundtables also provide a valuable forum for discussion and professional opinions on particularly timely and tricky ethical issues.

In this issue of the *Journal of Medical Speech-Language Pathology* we also encounter ethics and change. We have an excellent tutorial on ethics that was presented at a meeting of the Academy of Communication Disorders and Sciences by a professional with expertise and advanced degrees in both speech-language pathology and law. This is a perceptive and constructive essay entitled "The Language of Ethics in Clinical Practice." I am sure it will stand as a frequently cited and valuable resource for readers of our journal. In addition to this gem of a contribution, we present an update of the World Health Organization's Revised Classification in our Health Care Forum. We also have three articles on Parkinson disease, including research in articulatory kinematics, incidental learning and verbal memory, and laryngeal response to Apomorphine stimulation. Articles on semantic organization in traumatic brain injury and neurolinguistic function and cocaine abuse round out this issue.

On a more personal note, readers will notice that with this issue there is a new home of the editorial office of the *Journal of Medical Speech-Language Pathology*. I have accepted a position as the Francis Eppes Professor of Communication Disorders at Florida State University. Our journal must acclimate from its hospitable home among the saguaros and flowering cacti of Arizona State University in the Southwest desert to the dogwoods and Spanish moss-laden 100-year-old live oaks of Tallahassee near the beaches of the Gulf of Mexico. Change and ethics. And so it goes. Our friend Robert Frost reminds us not only of the ethereal flavor of life's changes, but also of the miles to go before we sleep.

REFERENCE

Frost, R. (1914). *North of Boston.* New York: Henry Holt and Co.

CHAPTER 33

LIGHT IN THE ATTIC

There is a light on in the attic.

—Shel Silverstein (1981)

" I had a stroke in 1995. I have aphasia. I see many of you asking for help. Work on your self every day. DON'T GIVE UP! . . . Things I do: Join a stroke club. I am in 3 clubs and help run one. Do volunteer work at your local hospital. If you can, get into the rehab section helping other stroke people . . ."

The advice in the quote above is contained in a posting in a chat room section of the website of the National Aphasia Association (156 Fifth Avenue, Suite 707, New York, NY 10010; http://www.aphasia.org). The NAA is an organization that promotes and provides awareness of aphasia and services to people who are challenged with the disorder. The NAA Pen Pal chat room section is a forum for people and families who are blindsided with the lightning like "strike" that leaves them with shattered communication. The forum provides a place to vent as well as a place for valuable information crafted by people who have been there and done that. The insider's perspective on aphasia and recovery is a theme that has appeared occasionally in both the professional and trade literature. The NAA has a nice selection of materials and publications that can he ordered at nominal cost to help people understand the condition. A previous issue of this journal (Vol. 2, No. 1, March 1994) presented the views of a professor of philosophy who had a stroke and developed some interesting ideas on the relationship between thought and language based on his own experience (Olson, 1994). Olson developed some interesting insights on thought and language and McNeil (1994) commented on his ideas in the same issue.

In this issue we have another perspective from the inside looking out. Drs. Nancy Kerr, a professor of Counseling and Rehabilitation Psychology at Arizona State University, and Barbara Lucelle, Ph.D., a speech-language pathologist, present some of the professional and personal reflections on their own recoveries from aphasia and their interpretation of some of the good, the bad, and the ugly relative to the therapy they received. Readers can unearth nuggets of wisdom from this uncommon view of aphasia and recovery. Also in plentiful supply in this trove are warnings, frank evaluations of what was not helpful, and several suggestions and ideas for generating empirical research and formulating testable hypotheses about intervention issues. One can see implications for the study of intervention and therapy that relate to service provision; setting, dose, task, and goal selection; task validation; and outcome measures, all issues that reside in the heart of any therapeutic procedure. We also see clinical lessons that relate to medical and social history and the mistakes that can be made from hasty assumptions created from casual observation. Dr. Kerr, for example, has a vision problem and uses a wheelchair, conditions that the casual historian might associate with her aphasia and stroke, until it is discovered that both of these conditions preceded her stroke.

Drs. Kerr and Lucelle are courageous in their disclosure of their impairments and the handicaps that accompanied their language compromise and are motivated to tell their stories because of their deep-rooted interest in the clinical process and in clinical teaching. I think this insider's point of view on therapy for aphasia is enlightening and inspiring. It should be required reading for all students who are faced with the sometimes overwhelming challenges of planning and implementing their first faltering steps down the path of becoming sensitive and educated aphasia clinicians.

Dr. Roberta Elman helps us out by presenting a useful commentary on this memoir by two professionals who experienced aphasia. Dr. Elman's clinical experience and work with models of service delivery is widely respected in aphasiology, as is her careful clinical research. She presents her interpretation of the insider's point of view.

Another feature of this issue, which will remain as a regular contribution in future issues of our journal, is the perspective of another expert in communication disorders, Carol Frattali, Ph.D., who is employed by the National Institutes of Health in Bethesda, Maryland. Carol will contribute her suggestions, ideas, and updates related to the delivery of services in communication disorders against the dynamic kaleidoscope of the contemporary health care scene. Her information, presented in a section entitled Health Care Forum, is sure to be a valuable source of information, solace, and strategic planning for those of us who are baffled and frustrated by whoever is twisting the kaleidoscope.

In addition, this issue of our journal contains a comparative study of cognitive-linguistic profiles of people with Down syndrome and Alzheimer's disease and a Clinical Note on alaryngeal speech utilization.

The late Shel Silverstein (1981, p. 7) wrote creative and insightful children's poems that had an appeal beyond the pediatric set. His metaphor of a light in the attic will resonate with familiarity to any clinician who has worked with people who have experienced the devastation of aphasia. How many times have we seen the light flicker? How many times have we experienced the reward of the recovery process from those first stages of flicker to the point of restoration of acceptable life quality after communication has been coaxed, facilitated, and nurtured?

There's a light on in the attic.

Though the house is dark and shuttered,

I can see a flickerin' flutter,

And I know what it's about.

There's a light on in the attic.

I can see it from the outside,

And I know you're on the inside . . . lookin' out.

This issue provides us with the unique privilege of two insiders who share with us their journey through the days of flicker to the point where their professional and personal experiences can be molded into a beneficial point of view for clinicians who deal with the shutters of aphasia. Thank you, Drs. Kerr and Lucelle, for sharing your light with us.

REFERENCES

McNeil, M. (1994). Comment on Carl W. Olson, Ph.D. "Thought and language: An aphasic's view from the inside looking out." *Journal of Medical Speech-Language Pathology, 2,* 87–88.

Olson, C. (1994). Thought and language: An aphasic's view from the inside looking out. *Journal of Medical Speech-Language Pathology, 2,* 79–86.

Silverstein, S. (1981). *A Light in the attic.* New York: Harper and Row.

CHAPTER 34

MORPHOLOGY AND THE RED PRIEST

On arriving in Venice, Robert Benchley immediately wired a friend,
Streets are flooded, please advise.

— R. E. Drennan, *Algonquin Wits* (1968)

Well, the streets *were* flooded. So was the Piazza San Marco during high tides after 4 days of rain. So was the first level of the remarkable Scuola Grande di San Giovanni Evangelista, the site of the 1999 Academy of Aphasia. Amid 14th century splendor including frescoes, elaborate ceilings, and huge canvases painted by Venetian masters and elaborately lighted statuary that dominated the great hall, members of the Academy of Aphasia gathered for their annual meeting. Sometimes it was difficult to keep one's eye on the anachronistic computer-generated slides when a slight glance to the right or left revealed centuries old captured scenes of glorification, betrayal, and ascension among throngs of cherubs.

The glory and grace of Venezia was a most magnificent setting for learning about the latest theoretical and neurolinguistic approaches to aphasia. As always, this organization and meeting focuses more on the puzzle and mystery of the disorder of aphasia than it does on the applied rehabilitative issues surrounding the handicap and disability of it. For those of us with an interest in both, that skewing has grown to be expected. Recognition of the matter of rehabilitation of people with aphasia must be sought elsewhere. But detailed attention to theoretic aspects of aphasiology was abundant at this meeting. A prime focus was on imaging and lesion studies of aphasia and local Italian researchers presented in-depth symposia on lessons from animal models; imaging studies related to attention, neglect, and sentence comprehension; and such intriguing and debatable topics as the role of Broca's area in language comprehension and processing. Researchers from Finland, The Netherlands, Australia, the United Kingdom, the United States, Belgium, France, Germany, and Slovenia gathered to present, question, clarify, and generate new ideas on how to go about solving the riddle of shattered morphosyntax and semantic activation.

Amid this heady deliberation members of the Academy took umbrella-protected opportunity to enjoy some of the marvels of the islands of Venice with its miles of canals plied by gondola, vaporetti, and water buses. This particular visit endured a lot of moisture and flooding of the squares and narrow passageways during high tides. Narrow, elevated wooden footpaths were laid on metal frames and tourists and residents alike squeezed carefully about their business with only occasional interlocked umbrellas (*umbrelli?*). Twice, this visitor observed off-balance stumbles from the narrow platforms into the rising canal water, both by well-dressed, middle-aged tourists. Only the recall that "gallows humor" or finding delight in the humorous misfortune of others as a reported characteristic of right cerebral hemisphere damage prevented the slip of a giggle.

Members of the Academy were also treated to a magnificent short concert by the local arrangement hosts of the meeting. Venice availed itself to other opportunities as well. On the first day of arrival, this visitor discovered that a concert would be held on the ensuing Friday evening in the Pieta, the church/orphanage/school where Antonio Vivaldi actually plied his trade for 40-odd years. Having been an admirer of the Red Priest, as Vivaldi was called either for his flaming red hair or penchant for wearing bright red vestments, this concert was a unique opportunity to hear a Venetian string group with harp-sichord perform *Il Quatro Stagioni,* the famous Four Seasons, in the actual venue where it was most likely composed. Antonio Vivaldi (1678–1741) taught voice, violin, and other instruments to orphan girls at the Pieta. Those under the Red Priest's tutelage presented regular public recitals with such skill that one legend holds that parents in Venice attempted to pass their daughters off as orphans so that they could be admitted to the Pieta and be taught by the master.

Although Four Seasons almost has become the wallpaper or elevator ambiance of classical music, here was a performance in a venue that made it easy to allow the mind to drift through time and linger momentarily on creative work that has withstood the erosion and changing styles of centuries. Perhaps those who labor with the study of morphosyntax and semantics and joust with the mystery of aphasia will be as fortunate.

Our inaugural issue for the year 2000 has a number of offerings designed to provoke thought and further study of aphasia and a variety of other topics as well. We begin with work from the University of Queensland on the role of subcortical structures in linguistic processing. In this article, Copland, Chenery, and Murdoch reveal persistent deficits in complex language function follow-ing dominant nonthalamic subcortical lesions. Stout, Yorkston, and Pimental follow with a study of discourse production in traumatic brain injury. Follow-ing that is a contribution from Brazil on auditory processing and language in Down syndrome. We then have two unique Clinical Notes. Marshall presents some ideas and challenges born of his seasoned years of clinical research on how to cope with adequate documentation of clinical change in today's envi-ronment of health care reimbursement. His ideas are provocative and useful. This is followed by presentation of interesting cases of atypical neurovascular disease, stroke, and aphasia by Hartman and Heun. The history and clinical course of two individuals are traced, one with Osler-Weber-Rendu syndrome and one with Moya Moya disease. Our readership is sure to discover new ideas and comforting truisms in this issue, just as members of the Academy of Aphasia did as they explored research on morphology and ventured up side canals to enjoy the fruits of the Red Priest.

REFERENCES

Drennan, R. E. (1968). *Algonquin wits.* New York: Holt.

Heller, K., & Marinelli, D. (1997). *Antonio Vivaldi: The Red Priest of Venice.* New York: Amadeus Press.

CHAPTER 35

TURN, TURN, TURN

Time has no divisions to mark its passage. There is never a thunderstorm or blare of trumpets to announce the beginning of a new month or year. Even when a new century begins, it is only we mortals who ring bells and fire off pistols.

—Thomas Mann, *The Magic Mountain* (1924)

Are we sufficiently numbed by millenium bells? Perhaps every December issue of every periodical this year will have a retrospective of the century. We are bombarded with retrospective. The media flame the frenzy to reduce, simplify, explain, or sound bite a thousand years of history. We are tempted to whimper, "All right, already. Let us slip gently into the good century."

The *Utne Reader* reminds us that the 20th century has been rough going (Walljasper & Spayde, 1999). Atomic weapons. Ethnic cleansing. Wars. Auschwitz. Deforestation. Junk mail. Profit obsessed privatization of health care that seems to focus more on "manage" than "care." Entire professions threatened by hasty and ill-formed policy. Mergers evolving into megaconglomerates. Ubiquitous corporate sponsorship of everything from sports events to public buildings and schools leading us ever closer to the eventual saturation where even the months of the year will have corporate sponsorship. Not a pretty picture.

Pessimistic reflection on a century perceived as half empty rather than half full can certainly lead to despair and depression. So we must be alert not to allow ourselves to wallow in the mud of a century of negatives. Along with the challenges is a thousand-year history of great strides in many fields. Advances in science, technology, and medicine are a few of the most palpable candidates. *Utne Reader* reminds us of some of the less obvious bits and pieces worth saving from the 20th century. How about crossword puzzles? Dr. Seuss? Ben & Jerry's Cherry Garcia ice cream? The zipper?

Perhaps a good millenial-philosophical exercise would be for us to reflect on some of these obvious and less obvious items worth saving in our particular professions as well. Much of that worth is in the ongoing efforts to teach, to remediate, and to understand those things that detract from optimal quality of life. This issue of our journal once again reminds us and energizes the struggle to continue to pursue these gracious objectives. In this issue we have an excellent tutorial on possible roles of the insula in speech and language processing by Bennett and Netsell. From Australia comes a critical evaluation of management protocols for tracheostomy decannulation. Constantinidou reports on interference and recognition memory in brain injury. Dagenais and colleagues use delayed auditory feedback to assess processing skills in speakers with Parkinson disease, and finally Cariski and Rosenbek present a clinical report on the effectiveness of the Speech Enhancer.

Another reason for optimism is a recently crafted affiliation of the *Journal of Medical Speech-Language Pathology* with the Academy of Neurological Communication Disorders and Sciences (ANCDS). This is an organization designed to promote quality service to persons with neurologic communication disorders. *JMSLP* will be the official journal of ANCDS and will serve as a forum for Academy information. We are proud of this mutually beneficial affiliation and look forward to a long and fruitful association with the Academy of Neurological Communication Disorders and Sciences. See this issue for information on the organization by Lee Ann Golper, Ph.D., BC-NCD, President of ANCDS.

Once again an interesting and informative collection of thought, research, and clinical analysis selected to guide our readers as they go about the process of engaging in the daily professional activities that have changed considerably since the beginning of the century. Gone are some of the practices that seem quaint and simplistic to us now. We should remind ourselves that our current levels of practice and research will seem just as quaint to those assessing the 21st century. Some sage from long ago noticed that the only thing constant is change. For every season, turn, turn, turn.

May the unknown changes of the new century provide you with fullfillment and satisfaction. Happy New Mill.

REFERENCES

Mann, T. (1924). *The magic mountain*. New York: Modern Library.

Walljasper, J., & Spayde, J. (1999, May/June). The 20th century: What's worth saving? *Utne Reader*, pp. 42–49.

CHAPTER 36

DICTIONARIES

As sheer casual reading material, I still find the dictionary the most interesting book in our language.

—Albert Jay Nock, *Memoirs of a Superfluous Man* (1943)

Samuel Johnson was a lexicographer, a wordsmith, a writer of dictionaries. He was also a bit of a curmudgeon. Traces of his irritation can be found in some of his definitions as well as in his not-so-subtle opinions. He self-deprecatingly described a lexicographer as "a writer of dictionaries, a harmless drudge."

Johnson was not above taking a poke at his rivals or at others with whom he was on less than neighborly terms. He once defined oats as — "a grain, which in England is generally given to horses, but in Scotland supports the people." However, he had a few good words for words throughout his amblings. His love of language was not contained and occasionally he would rhapsodize about language by such pronouncements as, "I am not so lost in lexicography as to forget that words are the daughter of the earth."

Johnson also had a few things to say about the art of the essay. He called it a loose sally of the mind; an irregular undigested piece, not a regular and orderly composition. So much for essayists. So let us sally forth and consider once again the world of words and of compilations of words. As professionals who study and depend on language, we take pleasure in perusing books on words and language, as well as in just thumbing through dictionaries. I agree with Nock. They make great casual reading material. Sometimes the plot of a dictionary is not very beguiling, and those of us who have studied narrative and the grammar of an adequate episode may be disappointed with mere compilations.

But the utility of a dictionary goes well beyond being on call as a trusty reference. One merely needs to leaf through the "big book," our pet name for the huge unabridged work that was a treasured "stand-up-at-the-wedding" gift from a friend and colleague (who is such an obsessive wordsmith or word addict that he sometimes has to look up words he himself has used). The dictionaries get thicker and thicker.

We have explosions of knowledge and mushrooming vocabulary. Lexical growth and change are apparent everywhere. Influences that expand and reshape our vocabulary include advances in science and technology, new forms and styles in the arts, fashion, and leisure activities. We were recently reminded of these changes during the data analysis and scoring responses from a written generative naming task for the category of "sports." Acceptable contemporary answers not included in the classic Battig and Montague (1969) norms are such contemporary endeavors as "snowboarding," "rollerblading," and "motocross." Other influences on the dynamism of language include broader cultural and social movements such as concern with the environment, the women's movement, and changing appreciation for ethnic and cultural differences.

Sometimes modifications of the great "isms" of society, such as racism and sexism, are shepherded and mollified by the words we use or better not use. Ageism is one of the last bastions of archaic attitude that still seems entrenched. Jokes and light banter about the accumulation of birthdays are rampant. Sexist jokes and blatant ethnic humor are still around, but much less public and more tempered by sensitivity than in years gone by. Not so with birthdays, however. Novelty stores do a brisk business selling black crepe paper, black-painted canes, and other "over-the-hill" accoutrements for birthday parties. We are so inundated with the thousands of media messages that implore us to conceal, cover, color, camouflage, hide, or surgically alter the visible signs of the natural aging process that it is nearly impossible to escape the subtext message of "young is good; old is bad."

But our language does indeed evolve. It is far from static. Browsing through a dictionary reminds us of traditional as well as contemporary lingo, and word lists are only a part of the "big book." In it we can discover charts, tables, and illustrations about the currencies of the world, hominid fossil skull bones, basic knots and hitches, types and shapes of leaves, and the phases of the moon. In addition, we can always perch on a new word such as "insessorial" and discover its meaning.

We have been reminded of dictionaries recently by a couple of incidents. One was the introduction of Singular Publishing Group's two new dictionaries for communication sciences and disorders. Ray Kent and Sadanand Singh have collaborated on an illustrated dictionary of speech-language pathology that contains over 4,000 terms. A companion illustrated volume has been released in audiology. In keeping with contemporary electronic trends, these compilations are available on CD-ROM or in print.

The other reminder of dictionaries and how our professional language has evolved was the perusal of the article titles in this issue of our journal. We have articles on radiation therapy for T1 glottic carcinoma, botulinum toxin injections for torticollis, electropalatographic assessment; discourse in intractable epilepsy; and cerebellar ataxia secondary to high-dose cytosine arabinoside toxicity. During my graduate school days, the previous sentence would have been as communicative as speaking to me in Old Church Slavonic. Times and terms change.

So enjoy this most enlightening issue. And take the time to visit your old friend the dictionary. You'll be surprised how she's changed.

REFERENCES

Battig, W. F., & Montgomery, W. E. (1969). Category norms for verbal items in 56 categories: A replication and extension of the Connecticut category norms. *Journal of Experimental Psychology Monograph, 80*(3), 1–45.

Johnson, S. *Dictionary* (Preface). London: Strahan & Livington.

Nock, A. J. (1943). *Memoirs of a superfluous man.* New York: Harper & Row.

CHAPTER 37

CULTURES

Culture may even be described simply as that which makes life worth living.

—T. S. Eliot, *Notes Towards a Definition of Culture* (1948)

A while ago we published some research on quality of life and visited the sometimes deeply philosophical issues of what constitutes acceptable life quality, wellness, or relative happiness. Our bias is that human communication, and particularly barriers to human communication, are profound factors in the equation. No need to attempt to advance that argument with the readers of this journal, for that truly would be preaching to the choir. We are firmly committed and in most cases have devoted our professional lives to the issues of advancing understanding and explanation of the myriad tangles that can hinder communication. At the heart of this as well is the daily clinical effort to scratch down these obstacles in the attempt to make life more bearable for those who have been dealt the hand of communication disability.

A thought that comes to mind is the universality of communication disability across the thousands of language systems and cultures that dot the planet. Culture can serve as a vital ingredient to life quality as well as to reaction to disability. Yet so many of us fail, I think, to appreciate the depths of cultural influence on our clinical and research decisions. Within most nationalistic boundaries one can encounter a *pistache* of cultures that swim and mingle within and without what could be considered the cultural mainstream.

Some years ago, while we were conducting research on the identification and prevalence of communication disorders in the underserved American Indian populations of our state of Arizona, we were confronted with the cultural inappropriateness of our language acquisition screening devices, which had been developed for middle class, urban Anglo populations. Naming zoo animals was difficult and inappropriate for the 3- and 4-year-old Navajo children although they had no trouble at all with horse, coyote, sheep, goat, dog, and the other animals within their experiential realm. Even some of our color naming tasks were inappropriate and had to be modified to include the earth tones and hues that were much more within the experience and lexicons of a people who live in a starkly beautiful world of creams, corals, browns, reds, and purples. Worlds of other examples exist, including the interpretation that in certain cultures a more fatalistic philosophy about illness, stroke, and aphasia make participation in rehabilitation programs by spouses and family members quite problematic.

Recently I had an opportunity to begin to appreciate some previously unexplored aspects of Asian culture in conjunction with participation in the First Asia-Pacific Conference on Speech, Language, and Hearing held at the University of Hong Kong. First, the conference itself was a genuine treat with a diverse program that included such wide-ranging topics as:

Vocalic duration characteristics in various types of Cantonese alaryngeal speech;

Impairment of lexical tone production in stroke patients with bilingual aphasia;

Perceptual, acoustic, and respiratory changes in post-pallidotomy patients;

Cross-language studies of error patterns in cleft palate speech using electro-palatography; Levels of processing and verbal memory in dementia;

Aphasia management in a linguistically diverse society

The organizers of this conference, Paul Fletcher and his associates at the University of Hong Kong, assembled a rich and diverse conference program including considerable focus on Asia-Pacific issues in human communication and its disorders.

Ample opportunity presented itself for one to be immersed in the culture of Hong Kong as well, with exposure to the rich variety of foods, social festivities, and holidays. By either great planning or good fortune, conference participants could observe the celebration of National Day, with its spectacular display of fireworks over Victoria Harbor, as well as some of the intriguing ritual of the Mid-Autumn Festival. The latter festivity commemorates the Mongolian Revolution of the 14th century where legend holds that the Chinese Emperor's wife suggested that Chinese autonomy and freedom from the occupying Mongolian forces only could be achieved by enlisting the support of the villagers and commoners. A message was sent to the populace inside a rich lotus and sesame seed duck egg-yolk-filled pastry, known thereafter as Mooncakes. The surreptitious message, not unlike the format of the little messages in fortune cookies, requested an uprising on the night of the full moon; and the villagers were to signal their compliance by hanging a red lantern. History tells us that the revolution was successful, and that the Chinese people gained freedom from the Mongolian forces. The event is remembered in each Mid-Autumn Festival by the distribution of Mooncakes, the hanging of lanterns, and assembly in the parks and commons to observe and greet the rising moon with lanterns, candles, and contemporary children's plastic lighted cartoon-character balloons ("Hello Kitty" was a popular cartoon icon). It was a beautiful and meaningful bit of Chinese culture that enriched the many naïve visitors who were unaware of it. Surely, that is what T.S. Eliot meant when he characterized culture as simply that which makes life worth living.

I purchased some of the Mooncakes so that I could share the story and a taste of the festival experience with students in one of my graduate seminars. Some, of course, were unsure of trying the culturally different duck egg Mooncakes, although most plunged in and seemed to enjoy them. This triggered a good discussion of cultural influences on the practice of speech-language pathology, as well as a diversion into some of the culture-bound barriers we face in experiencing culinary and other aspects of an unfamiliar way of life. Most of my students could not generate much enthusiasm or curiosity for sampling the fare at the traditional Chinese Snake Shops that I described and illustrated. In these shops the beneficial strength and healing power of snake soup or snake and noodles could be enjoyed after selecting your own delectable reptile from a cage or drawer. As culturally dissonant as this may have been perceived by contemporary American graduate students, I discovered that we have some culinary practices within our own culture that may appear as dissonant to others.

The August issue of the *Atlantic Monthly* has an interesting piece on the opening of squirrel-hunting season in several states, including Kentucky, where in recent years a number of diagnosed or suspected cases of Creutzfeldt-Jakob disease (CJD) (the degenerative neurological disorder similar in some ways to mad-cow disease) have been tentatively linked to the regional practice of eating squirrel brains either scrambled with eggs or in a stew. According to the August Almanac in the *Atlantic Monthly* (p. 10), from 1993 to 1997 physicians diagnosed 11 cases of CJD in rural west Kentucky. All the victims had a history of eating squirrel brains. While most cultural practices should be approached with an appreciation of context and without judgment, perhaps certain potentially dangerous culinary habits should be dished up with a warning. Unless one is willing to risk Creutzfeldt-Jakob disease perhaps Mooncakes would be a better choice than squirrel brains.

This issue of our journal has some cultural enrichment as well. We open with a descriptive piece on vibratory characteristics of the pharyngoesophageal segment in total laryngectomees by Dworkin and associates from the Wayne State University School of Medicine. Our second offering moves up the vocal tract to explore velopharyngeal function in subgroups of individuals with ALS from researchers in Canada. Marsha Zak presents some enlightening insights on what people in medical speech-language pathology know about brain tumors. Next, a study of attention in adolescents with brain injury is described by Robinson from Boston. A clinical note on treatment of spastic dysarthria with botulinum toxin A is presented by Lapco, Forbes, Murry, and Rosen of the Eye and Ear Institute at the University of Pittsburgh. We cap this issue with two book reviews. Leslie Gonzalez-Rothi reviews and comments on a book devoted to the neuropsychological assessment strategy of clock drawing. Finally, Baker and Seaver review Antonio Damasio's *Decartes' Error*. This review is a provocative and intellectually stimulating exploration into the historic and sometimes mystical world of dualism, the self, the metaself, thought and language, and the marvelous and continually puzzling interaction between brain and rest of the body. The review by Baker and Seaver is a deeply erudite work that goads our curiosity not only to consult Damasio's fascinating work but to revisit Cartesian issues as well. Consultation with other times and other cultures can serve us well. We think therefore we must.

REFERENCES

Anonymous. (1998, August). The August almanac. *The Atlantic Monthly,* p. 10.

Eliot, T. S. (1948). *Notes towards a definition of culture.* New York: Harcourt, Brace.

CHAPTER 38

AQUARIUS

. . . call back yesterday, bid time return.

—Shakespeare, *Richard II,* Act III

1969. The moon was in the seventh house. It was the dawning of the Age of Aquarius. A time of social and political upheaval in the United States and around the world. Those who were around and cognizant remember it well. Those who were yet unborn were destined to experience its influence years later, in history and politics, in science and technology, in music and popular culture. Violent fighting broke out in Northern Ireland between Protestants and Roman Catholics. Richard Nixon was inaugurated as the 37th president of the United States, only to be dogged by scandal and forced to leave office in disgrace. Terrorist bombs exploded in a Jerusalem market. (Any of this sound familiar?) Senator Edward Kennedy had a driving accident returning from a small island in Massachusetts. Hundreds of thousands of people in several U.S. cities demonstrated against the Vietnam War. Golda Meir became Israel's Prime Minister and DeGaulle resigned as President of France.

Late night leisure reading consisted of *Portnoy's Complaint, The Godfather, Naked Came a Stranger* (written as a jest by 24 journalists from a New York newspaper, it became a runaway best-seller). Tunes that floated through the air included numbers from "Summer of Love," at the Woodstock Music and Art Fair. Other hummable 1969 ditties included *A Boy Named Sue, Aquarius, In the Year 2525,* and Malipiero's opera *Gil Eroi di Bonaventura.* The visual arts celebrated *O! Calcutta!* and *Hair* on Broadway and the films *Midnight Cowboy, Easy Rider, Oh! What a Lovely War,* and *Butch Cassidy and the Sundance Kid.*

The world mourned the passing of Gabriel Chevalier, French novelist; Jack Kerouac, American wanderer; Rocky Marciano, American boxer; Sharon Tate, American actress; Dwight D. Eisenhower, Judy Garland, and Boris Karloff. It also observed the 300th anniversary of the death of Rembrandt.

In sports and daily life, the Sydney-to-Hobart sailing race was won by "Morning Cloud," skippered by Edward Heath; Prince Philip maintained that Britain's royal family would have to ask Parliament to increase the Queen's allowance; hurricane Camille devastated the Gulf Coast and rains in California caused mud slides that destroyed or damaged 10,000 homes; the Montreal Canadiens won the Stanley Cup; Rod Laver, the Australian tennis great now recovering from a stroke, won his second Grand Slam; and Wilt "the Stilt" Chamberlain led the National Basketball Association in rebounds for the 8th year out of the past 10. Representatives of 39 nations met in Rome to survey pollution of the seas, and trouser outfits "became acceptable" for everyday wear by women in some countries.

In science and technology, little would surpass the milestone of the world's first landing of a lunar module on the moon's surface and the subsequent small step of Astronaut Neil Armstrong. The Concorde, an Anglo-French supersonic aircraft, made its first test flight; and in Thailand a new species of swallow, the white-eyed river martin, was discovered. The United States took steps to ban the use of the pesticide DDT, and the Nobel Prize for Medicine and Physiology went to M. Delbruck, A. D. Hershey, and S. E. Luria for work on the genetic structure of viruses.

Against this backdrop, a significant milestone was about to occur in the clinical science of neuromotor speech disorders as well. The culmination of years of clinical experience and clinical research was about to be published by the *Journal of Speech and Hearing Research* that emanated from the Mayo Clinic in Rochester, Minnesota. In two seminal articles that were to prove catalytic for renewed interest and research in motor speech disorders, Darley, Aronson, and Brown outlined a rating and classification system designed to bring a semblance of order to the seeming chaos of the dysarthrias. These articles, one entitled "Differential Diagnostic Patterns of Dysarthria," and the other, "Clusters of Deviant Speech Dimensions in the Dysarthrias," spawned a classic clinical text entitled *Motor Speech Disorders*, published in 1975. A dog-eared and broken-spined copy of that green-covered work rests on my professional bookshelf and is used to this day. I suspect that like copies can be found in offices and archival collections throughout the world. The work of Darley, Aronson, and Brown changed our definitions, our thinking, and our clinical practice. The momentum of its influence is felt now nearly 30 years later, and although it has inspired much research and a few reviews, we are long overdue for a critical analysis of the unfolding of the clinical science of neuromotor speech disorders since that milestone year of 1969.

Enter Kent, Kent, Duffy, and Weismer. In this issue of our journal, we are gratified to devote an entire issue to a work that reviews, synthesizes, analyzes, and interprets the evolution of our understanding of the dysarthrias since Darley, Aronson, and Brown. Kent, Kent, Duffy, and Weismer's ambitious work reviews speech-voice profiles, related dysfunctions, and the considerable advances in our understanding of the neuropathology of the dysarthrias. This scholarly and tutorial synthesis is destined to take its place as another classic of explanation and understanding of the dysarthrias for the span of time from 1969 to 1999. We are most pleased to present this issue as a significant component of the state of the clinical science in neuromotor speech disorders. May the spirit of the holiday season allow you to call back the contributions, satisfaction, and joy of yesterday, as well as appreciate the dawning of the age of today.

REFERENCES

Grun, B. (1979). *The timetables of history: A horizontal linkage of people and events*. New York: Simon and Schuster.

Darley, F. L, Aronson, A. E., & Brown, J. R. (1969a). Differential diagnostic patterns of dysarthria. *Journal of Speech and Hearing Research, 12,* 249–269.

Darley, F. L., Aronson, A. E., & Brown, J. R. (1969b). Clusters of deviant speech dimensions in the dysarthrias. *Journal of Speech and Hearing Research, 12,* 462–496.

Darley, F. L., Aronson, A. E., & Brown, J. R. (1975). *Motor speech disorders*. Philadelphia: W. B. Saunders.

Shakespeare, W. (1971). *Richard II*. Oxford: Clarendon Press.

CHAPTER 39

PERSONAL ACCOUNTS

I have been one acquainted with the night.

—Robert Frost, "Acquainted with the Night"
West-Running Brook (1928)

The night is a powerful metaphor. It is the end of a long day's journey. It is that good something we do not go gently into. It is occasionally not fit for man nor beast. It is of tropical splendor or of tyranny. It is where the blues reside. Susan Sontag says that illness is the night side of life (1978). She contends that everyone holds dual citizenship in the kingdom of the well and the kingdom of the sick. Although we all prefer to use only the good passport, sooner or later each of us is obliged, at least for a spell, to identify ourselves as citizens of the night.

A fairly rich literature exists, particularly in the area of neurological disorders and aphasia, of personal accounts of night life. The National Aphasia Association has an extremely useful set of references and listings to advance awareness and information about aphasia on its website (www.aphasia.org). Included in the site is a listing of some personal accounts of stroke survivors. Some of the titles hint at some of the challenges and trials along the path of rehabilitation: *Portrait of Aphasia. Aphasia: My World Alone. Jumbly Words and Rights Where Wrongs Should Be: The Experience of Aphasia from the Inside. Up from the Ashes.* These, and many others through the years, have given us a view of the unique perspective of those who have experienced these conditions and survived.

Well-known persons, including several Presidents of the United States, have suffered strokes. The list of presidential stroke victims includes John Quincy Adams, John Tyler, Millard Fillmore, Andrew Johnson, Chester Arthur, Woodrow Wilson, and Franklin Delano Roosevelt. In fact, accounts of one of Woodrow Wilson's speeches seem to indicate that he suffered a stroke during the speech (Fields & Lemak, 1989). On September 25, 1919 in Pueblo, Colorado, Wilson had difficulty walking up steps leading to the Memorial Auditorium. His address to the large audience went smoothly for a while and then he began to falter:

> *Germany must never he allowed — (the stopped and was silent.) A lesson must be taught to Germany (He stopped and again stood still.) The world will never allow Germany — (He stopped again and was reported to appear confused. Finally he finished the speech, but upon completion the President began crying.) (Fields & Lemak, 1989, p.192)*

In this issue we have a remarkable personal account and interpretation of some of the aftermath of stroke as well. One of the world's leading experts in communication disorders and a member of our Editorial Consultant Board, Arnold E. Aronson, suffered a thromboembolic CVA in June of 1994. He has contributed to our journal an article entitled, Dysarthria, Crying, and Laughing in Pseudobulbar Palsy from Right Middle Cerebral Artery CVA: Overview and Personal Account. It gives me a great deal of pleasure to publish this beautiful and trenchant jewel of insight into the phenomenon of emotional incontinence. Surprising and useful conclusions emanate from this review and it is as scholarly as it is courageous. Thank you for sending this to us, Dr. Aronson. It provides a poignant and remarkably unique perspective of the issue.

This issue of our journal has a genuine international flavor. In addition to Aronson's contribution from the Mayo Clinic, Rochester, in the United States, we have an aspect of auditory word and sentence comprehension in Alzheimer's disease from the University of Haifa and the Rambam Medical Center in Haifa, Israel. We also present an interesting clinical note from the Department of Neurology at the University Hospital in Nijmegen, The Netherlands. Rounding out the issue are contributions from Hux and colleagues on synthetic and natural speech processing in adults with and without aphasia, and an article with clinical implications on rate reduction methods for improving speech intelligibility in dysarthric speakers with Parkinson's disease by Dagenais Southwood, and Lee.

The night has a thousand eyes. It is good that it also has some courageous reporters who have been acquainted with the night and are willing to enlighten the dark by sharing their personal accounts with us.

REFERENCES

Fields, W. S., & Lemak, N. A. (1989). *A history of stroke: Its recognition and treatment.* New York: Oxford University Press.

Frost, R. (1928). Acquainted with the night. *West-running brook.* New York: H. Holt.

National Aphasia Association. (1998). www.aphasia.org Sontag, S. (1978, January 26). Illness is the night-side. *New York Review of Books.*

CHAPTER 40

BAD SCIENCE–GOOD SCIENCE

*Man is a credulous animal, and must believe something; in the
absence of good grounds for belief, he will be satisfied with
bad ones.*

—Bertrand Russell, "Outline of Intellectual Rubbish"
Unpopular Essays (1950)

Dumbing down. We hear it and read about it at every turn, perhaps more these days than in the past. Reductionism, absurdity, oversimplification, and sound bites appear to be everywhere in contemporary society, particularly when popular culture attempts to translate science. Alien abductions, strange lights over Phoenix, UFO Roswellmania, miracle cures, or horrific new diseases pepper the media. Scary promos saturate local television transmissions, particulary during ratings or "sweeps" time.

> *"A new flesh-eating virus, for which scientists have no explanation, is spreading like wildfire! Film on Eyewitness News."*
> *Illegal weapon found in supermarket chicken. Are fowl arming themselves? Film at six.*

Shock headlines on alleged events such as spontaneous human combustion (SHC) become part of belief systems transmitted and embellished by nonscientist authors and journalists and by sensational electronic media that embrace and sell the paranormal. Many of the promulgators of these stories and beliefs engage in the logical fallacy called *argumentum ad ignorantium* ("arguing from ignorance") that usually utilizes the strategy of a shift in the burden of proof. "You can't find the cause, so therefore it must be spontaneous human combustion. Prove that it isn't."

Some media programming does attempt to present balanced, critical analysis of pseudoscience and the paranormal. The American TV series Scientific American Frontiers on PBS conducted evaluations of water dowsing, alien autopsy, handwriting analysis, and claims of unlimited energy sources. Established scientists led viewers along scientifically based explanations and interpretations of these seemingly paranormal or unexplained phenomena.

But it sometimes appears that the paranormalists are winning over the populace, and even some policy makers and legislators. Mainstream media smack of becoming tabloidized. Radio talk show and print publications laud the sensational and "unexplained" and have attracted a vast following of believers. Conventions devoted to psychic and UFO events live well and prosper.

A recent issue (and all issues for that matter) of *Skeptical Inquirer: The Magazine for Science and Reason* (1998, 22[2]) contains several provocative essays and articles on contemporary issues in the search for scientific literacy. An excellent conference report presented in the current issue of *Skeptical Inquirer* analyzes public attitudes toward science and potential paths to scientific literacy. Other eloquent pieces include an analysis of "the price of bad memories," by Elizabeth Loftus on the risks and validity of facilitating "repressed memories." Also in the issue is a marvelous interview with Martin Gardner, an eminent intellectual who for years contributed the column, "Notes of a Fringe-Watcher," for *Scientific American*. One of Gardner's classic columns entitled "Did Adam and Eve Have Navels," is reprinted as well. Another highlight is a trenchant essay by Richard Dawkins on "Science, Delusion, and the Appetite for Wonder," in which he argues that science is well qualified to feed our human need for wonder and the strange, and we need not go back to the dark age of superstition and unreason where every time you lose your keys you suspect poltergeists, demons, or alien abduction. This issue of *Skeptical Inquirer* and the collected archive of the periodical is a good source of information on science, anti-science, and preposterism.

Nor is the health care industry immune to the influences of reductionism and in some cases pseudo-science. Pilgrimages to treatment centers that promise cures for the terminally ill through magic elixirs of ground peach pits and lizard tails have outlived the polypharmacy heydey of Theophile Bonet in the 14th century, when it was a common practice to rub, sniff, or smear desperate patients with any concoction the imagination could create. Today, families continue to drain their savings and resources cure-shopping as they fly to far-off lands to seek the cure of a guru, psychic-surgeon, or miracle-worker.

The perception of significant erosion in the quality of health care delivery in the United States over the past decade or two has sounded the alarm among consumers. Health-consumer activist groups are becoming increasingly militant in their opposition to bottom-line driven medical reductionism that forces all individual cases into broadly driven diagnostic categories while capitating and sending home those who may benefit from continued treatment. "Quality of care" is a concept that may at long last be receiving as much attention as health care economics. We can only hope that health care is not unduly influenced by bad science, special interest agendas, and profit-driven hemianopsia.

This issue of the *Journal of Medical Speech-Language Pathology* contains no preposterism and a fair share of good clinical science. We begin with information on methods of science with an article entitled, "Clinical Trials and Their Application to Communication Sciences and Disorders," by Baum, Logemann, and Lilienfeld. This is followed by a methodological study of dysphagia assessment by McCullough, Rosenbek, Robbins, Coyle, and Wood.

Hopper, Bayles, and Tomoeda present an intriguing idea on the use of toys to stimulate communicative function in individual's with Alzheimer's disease. Colleagues from London report their findings on psychological function in spasmodic dysphonia before and after botulinum toxin treatment. Cautions regarding orientation testing and responses are offered by colleagues from near the San Francisco peaks in Arizona, and finally, we reprint a clinical note by Ronald W. Netsell that considers the respiratory and velopharyngeal systems in speech rehabilitation for people with unintelligible speech and dysarthria.

Once again, this issue offers our readers data-based articles, clinical notes, and carefully drawn opinions on a variety of topics germane to medical speech-language pathology. We are indeed credulous animals, and this number of our journal offers credible science and good grounds for belief . . . along with an open invitation to our readership for skeptical analysis and interpretation.

REFERENCES

Russell, B. (1950). Outline of intellectual rubbish. *Unpopular Essays.* New York: Simon and Schuster.

Skeptical Inquirer: The Magazine for Science and Reason. (1998), 22(2).

CHAPTER 41

EGGHEADS

Oh, what a tangled web do parents weave
When they think their children are naïve.

—Ogden Nash, *The face is familiar* (1940)

Once again it is time to share some of the insights of my third grade student-friends who attend Kyrene de los Cerritos Elementary School in the shadow of South Mountain in Phoenix, Arizona. Each year I look forward to interacting with this group when their remarkable teacher presents units on health and handicap awareness. Again this year they wanted to learn about the brain and the types of disabilities and handicaps that can accompany brain damage. I took the opportunity to incorporate a little advocacy for ways to prevent brain damage, particularly by wearing a helmet during bicycling, skateboarding, and roller blading.

Pediatric head injury is a growing problem in many countries. Research by the Arizona Governor's Advisory Council on Spinal and Head Injuries revealed some surprising and alarming statistics regarding this phenomenon in our state. A significant portion of emergency room visits are devoted to pediatric head injury. Motor vehicle accidents lead the list of causes of traumatic cerebral ravage. Despite these frightening and persuasive data, in our state we still retain the archaic notion that the government has no right to restrict personal freedom by requiring motorcyclists to wear helmets. In a state with a significant rural population we also allow unrestrained children to ride in the back of pickup trucks and each year families are visited with tragedy when kids fly out of pickup truck beds or are victims of roll-over accidents. A surprising aspect of the epidemiologic study of head injury hospital admissions was the revelation that a significantly increasing number of pediatric head injuries are the result of falls from school playground equipment. (How about a soft landing zone around jungle gyms rather than concrete or tarmac?) Skate boards, roller blades, scooters, all-terror-rain vehicles, and bicycles also contribute startling aggregates to these data.

The Arizona Governor's Advisory Council on Spinal and Head Injuries has instituted a remarkable educational program to educate and inform, and perhaps to have an influence on these deadly trends. Many of us on the Council instituted programs of personal involvement in some of the educational efforts. My visits to Cerritos Elementary School were begun by the impetus of the Governor's Council and are sustained by the belief that perhaps a few emerging attitudes can be shaped. Also, it is a great opportunity to get reacquainted with the honesty of children and the realization that third-graders are not all that naive.

My most recent visit rewarded me once again. The questions continue to be insightful ("If a rattlesnake bites you on the big toe, how does the poison get all the way to the brain?"). The format of a group of wide-eyed school children sitting on the floor around you and continualy popping up with questions that seemingly burst from their mouths is a nice change of pace from university graduate students who on occasion show all of the enthusiam of a small soap dish.

During the most recent visit, I decided to attempt a minor demonstration on the role of helmet protection on fragile contents. To do this I brought several raw eggs, a magic marker, some tape, and some little helmet-like devices cut out of egg cartons. With great drama I explained first the nature of the protection of the skull, but that it sometimes was not sufficient, and that some added protection might help. We then drew facial features, named the likeness "Mr. Egghead," and proceeded to drop him on newspaper from a height of about three feet. Splat. Point made. Almost ... The next step was to try it again with protection, so facial features and curly hair (the girls in the group requested that we name this one "Ms. Egghead") were drawn on the second egg. The portion of egg carton faux helmet was carefully taped on. Ms. Egghead was elevated and dropped, and bounced intact. No yolk. Applause. Point completed.

Let me share with you once again some of the unique and unedited comments received in the form of illustrated thank you notes from this remarkable group.

I really liked it when we where talking about Mr. Egghead. Now I always where my helmet.

—Sinserly, Christian

Thank you for coming into our class and teaching us about the Brain. I learned about the white cord at the bottem.

—Sincerily, Alex

I really like you coming hear. I like learning about the brane. I learned that the brane controls the body.

—Sincirly, Daniel

It was excited when you dropt Mr. Egghead and he spater on the flor.

—Love, Ronell

Thank you for coming in to teach us about the brain. We learned a lot about parts of the brain like the cerrobellum.

—Alex A.

We learned lots of importent parts of our lover brain.

—Jeremiah

Thank you for the very fun and faceanayeding time here at Cerritos. The front of the brain looks like Elvis's hare.

—Danny

I learned a lot about the brain and alwees where your helmet, defenetly. Cool.

—Ali

I loved Mrs. And Mr. Egghead. I loved looking inside of the brain.

—Love, Rebecca

Thank you for coming to our class. I learned about the different stuff like the hipp campus.

—Brooks

My favrite part was when you twice a brain apart.

—Your friend, Caitlin

Dear Dr. LaPointe,
Why did Mr. Egghead have to die?

—Sinserly, Dane

Because he was not wearing his helmet, Dane. I hope all of you wear yours. Ogden Nash was right. We underestimate children when we characterize them as naive. They may be still learning to spell, but most of them surely get the point. Perhaps when some of them grow up to be legislators they will remember early lessons and realize that enlightened public policy can influence health and safety of the citizenry.

This issue of our journal has a variety of topics of interest. We start with an article on the effects of speaking rate on word recognition in Parkinson's disease and normal aging by researchers from Indiana University. Next we feature a critical look at severity classification measures and subject criteria in studies of mild pediatric traumatic brain injury by Lustig and Tompkins. Lewin and LaPine present a study of intraluminal pressure in patients with tracheoesophageal and trahceojejunal puncture, followed by a clinical note on the role of physical therapy in multidisciplinary treatment of muscle tension dysphonia. Lastly, we present two book reviews: one of Jean-Dominique Bauby's remarkable book The diving bell and the butterfly; and then an opinion on clinical neurophysiology of attention.

We hope this issue provides you with information and inspiration.

REFERENCE

Nash, Ogden (1940). *The Face is Familiar.* Garden City, NY: Garden City Publishing Co.

CHAPTER 42

LIVES

Biographies are but the clothes and buttons of a man—the biography of the man himself cannot be written.

—Mark Twain, *Autobiography* (1924)

A s with so many of his pithy insights, Twain once again directs us to examine certain assumptions about life, truth, and, in this particular case, the fallibility of biography. Even the most seemingly complete and voluminous attempt to net the essence of a person's life is doomed to omit much from the capture. Surely, nuances of one's personality or history would be easy to miss against the backdrop of the limitless number of events to highlight. Although subtleties of a life might be understandably overlooked, sometimes significant activities and even momentous contributions to humanity may go unrecognized, unidentified, or hidden by the protective coloration of later achievement. Consider, for example, the following descriptions and quotes excerpted from a celebrated scientist's biography and play the game of trying to guess who it is:

> *Cancer is characterized by the presence of an element without analogy in the body economy; this deserves to be termed the cancerous element.*
>
> *If it is true that the monsters often are degraded organisms which in some of their parts repeat the features and dispositions of types belonging to a lower rung of the ladder, one may say without exaggeration that cancer is a pathological monstrosity.*
>
> *[This man] and Redfern in Edinburgh, independently but simultaneously, reversed the old Hippocratic idea that cartilage was as dead as hair and nails.*
>
> *Not all deformed feet were the result of disease, and two or three 18th Century authors [along with this scientist] had drawn attention to the injuriousness of shoes.*
>
> *While many of these instruments are no longer in use, some have been re-invented, and [this man's] goniometer, osteometer, osteometric board, dynamometer, and sliding-spreading calipers have undergone only minor changes.*
>
> *The only way out is to admit evolution and transformation as a necessary consequence to the way in which species have been distributed and constituted in history.*
>
> *In 1861 . . . [this man] set up a modest experiment with cornflowers (bachelor buttons or blue bottles) in his garden.*
>
> *[This man's] friends from the two Chambers of Parliament celebrated his election as a Senator with a banquet at the customary gala hotel.*
>
> *He made a cult of his duties [and] burdened his shoulders out of all proportion . . . the curtains of his study were saturated by cigar smoke, [and] . . . according to one of his granddaughters, "these feverish movements of the man for whom there will [never] be enough time to bring forth all that fermenting, boiling life trying to take shape within. [He] knows this and drives himself to crowd several lives into the one that is too short.*

So who is this eminent scientist whose contributions and attributes are extolled in the above descriptions and quotations? Cancer researcher, biologist, anthropologist, professor, politician ... Enough clues? You are absolutely right. The man described above is Pierre Paul Broca, born on June 28, 1824 in the village of Sainte-Foy-la-Grande, France and known above all for his remarkable case studies, published in 1861, on the "seat of articulate language" in the brain. Much of the breadth of his work is unrecognized or overshadowed by the celebrity he achieved in neuroscience and by the subsequent naming of that imortant cortical landmark as "Broca's area."

These descriptions and quotations about Broca's life are all taken from a remarkable biography entitled, *Paul Broca: Explorer of the Brain*, by Francis Schiller. The many facets reflecting a life are no more evident than in Schiller's study of Broca, and we grow to appreciate much more about the man than myopic recognition of only his renowned case studies of Leborgne and Lelong.

In this issue of our journal we present biography and case study as well, along with empirical studies and survey research. This issue is remarkably variegated. From Harvard, Verdolini and Palmer describe a "Profiles" approach to voice assessment. Kent and associates present a fascinating case report of atypical palilalia, a disorder of speech fluency so under-recognized and infrequently studied that we wonder what typical might be. Next, from London, Papathanasiou and colleagues present a survey study of perceived stigma in individuals with spasmodic dysphonia. This is followed by a study of ventilator-supported communication by Isaki and Hoit and a meticulous clinical note on the use of biofeedback rehabilitation of speech breathing by our colleagues near the Great Barrier Reef—Thompson-Ward, Murdoch, and Stokes.

Finally, Dr. Eelco Wijdicks from the Mayo Clinic, Rochester has reviewed for us the biography of another famous French neurologist, Charcot. A contemporary of Broca, and considered one of the pillars of the French school of Neurology, Charcot achieved much of his fame for serving as the mentor and teacher of so many other neuroscientists destined for greatness. These glimpses into lives and history can give us insight into the foundations of a clinical science and allow us to value the clothes and buttons of our predecessors. May the melange of this issue along with the spirit of the season suffuse you with joy and enlightenment.

REFERENCES

Schiller, F. (1992). *Paul Broca: Explorer of the brain*. Oxford, UK: Oxford University Press.

Twain, M. (1924). *Autobiography*. New York: Harper & Brothers.

CHAPTER 43

DAYS-DAZE

What are days for?
Days are where we live.
They come, they wake us
Time and time over.

—Philip Larkin, *The Whitsun Weddings* (1964)

S ome days are better than others. Some days beget rude surprises. . . . a firm grasp of the obvious about life. As the American humorist Ogden Nash is alleged to have remarked, "Life is not having been told that the man has just waxed the floor."

These surprises serve to remind us to relish and luxuriate in the days that are good. Reflection and introspective savoring behavior can get veiled and neglected in the daily shuffle, but these are good practices to instill into our regular routine. Events preceding and subsequent to the recent Clinical Aphasiology Conference (CAC) in Bigfork, Montana have underscored the wisdom of appreciating the unsullied days. And this annual conference is surely among those days that we mark as excellent. The CAC has now been held for 27 years and is a gathering of people who are very concerned not only with an understanding of the disorder of aphasia but an acknowledgement and consideration of people with aphasia. I have had the pleasure, after missing the inaugural meeting fathered by Bruce Porch in the basement of the Albuquerque VA Hospital, of attending 26 of these conferences in a row. This annual meeting never fails to satisfy in both professional enhancement as well as in the realm of socialization with newcomers and long-time friends who share a genuine interest in the handicap and disability of aphasia.

This year's CAC was held in the environment of the Flathead Lake Lodge on the shore of one of the largest natural lakes in the Rocky Mountains and close by the majestic Glacier National Park and the intriguing Two Medicine country of the American author Ivan Doig. The scenery, recreational opportunities, and Dude Ranch flavor of this setting were in keeping with the long tradition of the CAC to find a place where we can have some fun as well as learn. A sampler of his year's program, Chaired by Brenda Adamovich, included such topics as:

Predicting lifestyle satisfaction of young chronically aphasic adults;

Verb preference effects in sentence comprehension;
    Longitudinal changes in aphasic discourse;

Effects of training multiple form classes of word retrieval;

Progressive treatment of primary progressive aphasia;

Predictors of change in children and adolescents following TBI;

Effects of targeting sound groups in treatment of apraxia of speech;

Access versus degraded store deficits in naming disorders in aphasia and Alzheimer Disease

Many other useful and interesting papers were presented including an introspective series of round table discussions on a variety topics *(Specialty recognition and board certification; Right hemisphere damage; Dementia; Apraxia of speech; Social approaches to treatment; Computer applications; What graduates need to know about neurogenic communication disorders in the 21st century; and Use of on-line measure of MRI, eye movements, and evoked potentials).* A special session was conducted as well on *The impact of changing times on neurogenic communication disorders.* Essays and reviews along with heated and enlightened discussion focused on managed care, service delivery in the private sector and in the VA Medical Centers, academic curricula, and research, as well as on introspective analysis of *Social Darwinism and change in the Clinical Aphasiology Conference.*

The invited guest speaker this year was the internationally recognized expert on episodic memory, Dr. Endel Tulving. His trenchant information, as well his accessibility for informal discussion and immediate integration into the warmth and spirit of the CAC, was added value.

This fruitful program was only enhanced by the well-deserved reputation of the CAC for revelry and recreation and ample informal discussion of real-life clinical problems. This year, as seems to be increasing annually, we had participation from international colleagues. Friends from Canada, Germany, Japan, and Australia contributed to the perspective and enriched social melange of the meeting.

An international flavor is apparent as well in this issue of our journal. Once again our prolific colleagues from Down Under contribute by informing us about interlabial pressure during performance of speech and nonspeech tasks as well as a technical note from an interdisciplinary team of engineers and speech-language pathologists on the implications of viscosity and density of fluids used for dysphagia assessment. We present as well a study of the effect of Parkinson's disease on language by a group from the University of Arizona; a study of aphasic adults' knowledge of goal-directed action categories; and an analysis of word association behaviors of survivors of severe traumatic brain injury.

So we wish you some informative moments as you peruse this issue of our journal and remind you to take advantage of the rich opportunities for professional and social fortification offered by conferences and meetings of your peers. The CAC is one such meeting that blends science, clinical insights, and this year, bountiful cowboy-flavored socialization with good friends.

What are days for? Days are where we live. You are gently reminded to take some time to enjoy these days because you never know when someone will wax the floor.

REFERENCE

Larkin, P. (1964). *The Whitsun weddings.* New York: Random House.

CHAPTER 44

ROTTEN REVIEWS

Heller wallows in his own laughter and finally drowns in it. What remains is a debris of sour jokes, stage anger, dirty words, synthetic looniness, and the sort of antic behavior the children fall into when they know they are losing our attention.

—Review in *The New Yorker* of Joseph Heller's *Catch-22*

Just about anyone who has written professionally knows the sting of an unsympathetic review. Even in the wondrous world of academic and professional publishing, we must endure and reconcile opinions of our work that others regard as less than perfect — or as drivel. The editor's dilemma is the quandary faced when esteemed peer reviewers come to opinions on a manuscript that are at the opposite ends of the continuum. Fortunately, this does not happen often, at least in my experience, and this rarity can be attributed to the skills and expertise of the Editorial Consultant Board and the ad hoc reviewers who handle the chores of manuscript evaluation. But once in a while it happens. And it did with one of the manuscripts in this issue. One reviewer thought that the submission was one of the cleanest, most cogent pieces of work he had ever seen, and in fact suggested that it might be published "as is" with little or no revision. The other reviewer took a different stance and suggested that the very same manuscript was replete with biased subjectivity, unwarranted inference, and even questioned the motivation of the authors.

When this kind of diversity of opinion is received on the very same manuscript, the editorial staff has several options. These include siding with one reviewer or the other to tip the balance or sending the work out for further review to try to achieve a consensus. Whatever the decision, the peer review process works and it can be trusted to generate reasonably sound opinions on whether or not manuscripts contain fatal flaws, unresolved threats to internal or external validity, or in fact may be stellar contributions that will not disintegrate in the dusty boneyard of forgotten esoteric ramblings, but will live on to instruct, elucidate, and perhaps inspire yet unborn writers and researchers to add to the accumulating pool of what we know about our world. The peer review process is quite sacred in the scientific world and separates the claims of clinical science from the easily biased worlds of anecdotal evidence, testimony, and attempts to con, persuade, or sell. Psychic hotlines, miracle cabbage diets, and abblasters may have their place in the universe, but their claims to superiority are frequently far removed from what constitutes adequate evidence.

But even the famous and stalwarts of the world of science and literature have had to endure rotten reviews. A few examples:

From a review of Ernest Hemingway's *The Sun Also Rises*:

> *His characters are as shallow as the saucers in which they stack their daily emotions . . .*

From a review of Shakespeare's *Hamlet*:

> *It is a vulgar and barbarous drama, which would not be tolerated by the vilest populace of France or Italy . . . one would imagine this piece to be the work of a drunken savage.*

On Walt Whitman's *Leaves of Grass*:

> *Whitman is as unacquainted with art as a hog is with mathematics.*

All of these reviews are contained in a marvelous little compilation entitled *Rotten Reviews* (1987), edited by Bill Henderson. Anyone who has despaired of unseemly opinions of their written work can gain solace by keeping this small gem handy.

And with this issue we instigate a new feature in our journal. We will periodically review books, tests, or materials in our field that we feel our readership finds useful. Penelope S. Meyers, Ph.D., has been selected to serve as our Book Review Editor, and she will call on a stable of literate professionals to offer opinions about available publications. This month an interesting book on amyotrophic lateral sclerosis is reviewed by Edythe Strand, Ph.D. Along with this inaugural review are articles on psychogenic stuttering by contributors from the Mayo Clinic, Rochester; a survey of communication assessment protocols for children with traumatic brain injury; a clinically relevant article from Swedish colleagues on speech modification in multiple sclerosis; and a study of expiratory muscle conditioning in speech-impaired children.

REFERENCE

Henderson, B. (Ed.). (1987). *Rotten reviews: A literary companion*. New York: Penguin Books.

CHAPTER 45

MENTORS

I have never let schooling interfere with my education.

—Mark Twain

One thing about education is that sometimes the schooling allows one to find a mentor or two. And then schooling and education are truly paddling down the same stream. At our university since 1987 the Graduate College and Arizona State University Foundation have recognized the value of this process by honoring exceptional graduate mentors. Outstanding mentors are nominated and selected and then publicly recognized for the role they have played in the lives of past and present students.

In Homer's *Odyssey,* Mentor was the loyal advisor of Odysseus entrusted with the care and education of Telemachus. As with so many words and concepts from classic Greek origin, therein springs our present day notion of mentor. The *Random House Unabridged Dictionary* suggests that a mentor is a "wise and trusted counselor or teacher." It also lists Mentor as a town in Northeast Ohio, but I think the first definition is the appropriate choice.

As Bianca Bernstein stated in a brochure honoring outstanding Arizona State University mentors, the ephemeral nature of mentoring defies precise definition, but it is clear to most that it goes well beyond the traditional teaching role. Bernstein states, "In addition to teaching, a mentor guides. Beyond merely listening, a mentor understands. A professor cares, a mentor invests. A professor tells, a mentor shows. A professor connects, a mentor bonds. A professor nurtures, a mentor cradles. A professor gains respect, a mentor gains admiration and lifelong association."

Most of us can point to an extremely influential teacher or two who went beyond the "learning objectives" of the course and transcended the syllabus of their curriculum assignments to genuinely assume the cloak of "mentor." Maybe the most distinguishing and flattering aspect of mentorship is what Bernstein calls the role of "identity model." A real mentor ushers the student through the process of becoming socialized to the values, norms, practices, and attitudes of a discipline. This does not exclude the development of friendship.

Mentors of influence in my education include not only Mrs. Kurth, who showed us societies and cultures beyond the swamps of Channing, that tiny railroad town in the Upper Peninsula of Michigan (and accompanied us ice skating and on field trips to museums and libraries in neighboring counties), but also professors who in the more traditional mentoric sense guided and befriended us within the profession. Ned Welcome Bowler was the sterotypic pipe-fiddling, Harris-tweed wearing professor at the University of Colorado who made us think, did not suffer mediocrity without incisive critique, and prodded us to evaluate all angles on the prism of complex issues.

Also at the University of Colorado, another lifelong mentor and friend showed up on the scene. Robert Terry Wertz took his first job as an assistant professor, fresh out of Stanford, and brought expertise in neurogenic communication disorders, an abundance of patience and good humor, and a dollop of inspiration to graduate students emerging from their cocoon of naivete. Jay Rosenbek and I benefited greatly from Wertz's mentorship and have maintained a 30-year friendship with him that has included not only co-authored writing, but also softball games against the enormous, more physically gifted and dreaded goons of the Public Service team. He also participated with us in cassoulet and wine, goofy parlor games of Charades, a 30-year exchange of good books and music, and countless discussions over some good and some not so good servings of broiled fish on the state of the profession, the real nature of apraxia, and whatever happened to Terrance Stamp.

At the recent American Speech-Language-Hearing convention in Seattle, Wertz was given the highest award afforded by our professional association, the Honors of the Association. Those of us in the audience who saw his professional life reviewed agreed with the recorded comment of a friend, "Your memorable influence will continue in the people you have nurtured and who now can try to pass it on with your style and grace."

In this issue of the journal we have another outstanding example of a mentor—one who has had profound influence on the contemporary generation of aphasiologists. Dr. Harold Goodglass is featured in a "Conversation" conducted by Dr. Nancy Helm-Estabrooks. Goodglass has been feted many times over in recent years, not the least of which was the naming in his honor of the Harold Goodglass Aphasia Research Center in Boston. He is one of the true giants in the study of aphasia, and he has produced an impressive number of progeny. A collection of articles by former students and professional colleagues published in his honor in the journal *Aphasiology* (1988, Vol. 4, No. 4/5) provided ample evidence of his research influence. In our conversation with Harold Goodglass, we see some more personal facets, including mentors and professionals who influenced him. We felt our readers would enjoy and appreciate this conversational visit with a contemporary authority in aphasiology.

Also in this issue, we have a novel approach to group treatment in aphasia by Jan Avent, which uses concepts from cooperative learning models. We have an article that emanated from the Mayo Clinic, Rochester, on ataxic dysarthria that questions the homogeneity of this disorder, and an interesting and timely survey on post-Master's degree education in adult medical speech-language pathology by Shadden and colleagues from Arkansas. We conclude with a clinical note on voice characteristics following radiation therapy in subjects with glottic cancer.

Although this issue cannot take the place of a good mentor in professional development, perhaps it will supplement the benefit provided by that cadre of mentors past and those still to come. Mark Twain had a lot of cogent observations about life and about education. Leave it to him to imply that much of the value of a genuine education is not merely in the schooling itself, but in the richness of the mentor relationships that are nurtured and extend into mutually fulfilling collaborations way beyond pomp and circumstance. So thank you to Ned, to Terry, to Harold, to the ice-skating Mrs. Kurth, and to all teachers who embrace the true spirit of the ancient Greek Mentor.

REFERENCE

Bernstine, B. (1996). *Outstanding Graduate Mentors*. [Brochure.] Tempe: Arizona State University Graduate College and ASU Foundation.

CHAPTER 46

QUALITY

For life is joy, and mind is fruit,
And body's precious earth and root.

—John Masefield, *The Everlasting Mercy* (1930)

Q uality of life is elusive. Not only is it difficult to determine whether or not satisfying life quality has been attained, but the actual definition of acceptable quality of life is slippery. "On the balance, more pleasure than pain," is the simplest ledger some anonymous philosopher created to help us measure a happy life. But there is more to it than that. Each of us knows whether or not our life has been worth it, and the criteria for this determination are cultural, societal, and highly individualistic.

Quality of life includes the ability to participate in life's offerings and activities and to derive satisfaction from them. Most of us feel that health and disease play a major role in this determination. More to the point, since few of us run the gamut unscathed, is how we cope or deal with the inevitabilities of unwellness. An individual's wishes, expectations, goals, dreams, limitations in achieving these phantasms, as well as each peculiar value system are all critical factors that color our conclusions about life.

Piqued by the topic and impressed enough with the innocence and veracity of the opinions of my friends in the third grade at Kyrene de los Cerritos Elementary School, once again, through the good graces of their most competent and caring teacher, I asked their opinion on the quality of life. The question was something like, "What makes a good life? What are the things in your life that make it a good life?" As usual, their answers are enlightening and trenchant.

MEGAN'S LIST	*dance, food, reading, rain, vegies, pencils, and fruit*
ELISE'S LIST	*parents, weddings, computers, and swimming*
CARI'S LIST	*candy, pajamas, pets, hair, breakfast, and summer break*
HARRISON'S LIST	*friends, food, drinks, home, clocks, animals, silverware, language, and movies*
TAYLOR'S STATEMENT	*The Phoenix Suns dancers are my babysitters.*
NICK'S LIST	*my dog, my fish*
DEVIN'S (UNEDITED)	*Playing baseball as a kid. Playing with my baby cosin.*
BEN'S LIST	*Having ice cream. Being alive.*
JESSICA'S STATEMENT	*The thing that makes my life good are my friends because if I didn't have any friends I wouldn't be happy. All I would be doing is nothing around the house.*

These are the opinions and some of the determinants of life quality by children at one school in the foothills of the South Mountain in Arizona. Many academics and clinicians also are interested in the questions surrounding determinants of satisfactory life quality. At our university, Morris A. Okun has devoted much of his research effort to the discovery of perceptions of wellness.

M. P. Lawton also has studied life quality, particularly the role of environmental factors and other aspects of well-being in older people (Lawton, 1983, 1991). Some researchers have developed health surveys and medical outcomes measures that incorporate opinions within the domains of physical functioning, role limitations, social functioning, bodily pain, mental health, vitality, ambulation, body care, communication, home management, recreational and social interactions, and employment. Nevertheless, controversy continues over the ability to define quality of life, let alone measure it validly and reliably. The concept is of sufficient consequence to assure that rumination and research will continue.

And in this issue it does. We begin Volume 4, Number 4 with an excellent study of the effect of voice disorders on the quality of life. This work comes to us from a team of researchers at the University of Iowa and connects the existence of voice disorders with perceptions of diminished quality of life by those who have endured phonatory and laryngeal aberrations. This is the kind of research that may help convince third party payers, managed care administrators, capitators of rehabilitation services, and other bottom-line bursars who continue to lacerate health care benefits that cognitive and communicative disorders are critical to an individual's sense of well-being. Voice and speech are not frills. They are what make us human and help distinguish us from the iguanas. As is evidenced by this fine article, disorders of these functions can be devastating to life quality and need to be viewed and valued as important.

An article by King and Hux follows on attention in adults with and without aphasia. More and more attention is being directed, with only partial pun intended, to the nature of the control of information processing and particularly the effects of both left and right hemisphere lesion on attention and their impact on language use. This article continues the pursuit of understanding on attention and aphasia that has been previously visited by researchers at the University of Pittsburgh, Arizona State University, the University of Iowa, and elsewhere. Also in this issue is an article that reveals other characteristics of individuals with aphasia. In this work, by Tina Smith, metalinguistic judgments of people with Broca's aphasia are investigated.

Two fine clinical notes complete this volume. First, Murdoch and Lethlean describe language dysfunction in Binswanger's disease, lending additional evidence to the notion of subcortical participation in language. Also, Leiter and Windsor, in a note that contains many concrete clinical suggestions, report on compliance of geriatric dysphagic patients with safe-swallowing instructions.

So here is another well-rounded and informative issue for those who toil in the fields of medical speech-language pathology. May you continue your labor with satisfaction and also have the opportunity to enjoy some determinants of what constitutes a rewarding quality of life. In this special season, here's wishing you friends, reading, pets, ice cream, dance, drinks, and language. For life is joy, and mind is fruit.

REFERENCES

Lawton, M. P. (1983). Environment and other determinants of well-being in older people. *The Gerontologist, 23,* 349–357.

Lawton, M. P. (1991). A multidimensional view of quality of life in frail elders. In J. E. Birren, J. E. Lubben, J. C. Rowe, & D. E. Deutchman (Eds.), *The concept and measurement of quality of life in the frail elderly* (pp. 3–27). New York: Academic Press.

Masefield, J. (1930). *The everlasting mercy.* New York: Macmillan.

CHAPTER 47

STRIKES

... Today .... I consider myself ... the
luckiest man on the face of the earth.

—Lou Gehrig, Yankee Stadium, July 4 (1939)

With his typical spirit and battler mentality, Lou Gehrig responded to the cheers and tears of a packed Yankee Stadium, a scene immortalized on Hollywood celluloid, with positivism and hope. Lou Gehrig was a classic American baseball player, back before the era of spoiled, overindulged athlete heroes, who quietly became known as the "Iron Horse" for playing in 2,130 consecutive games, hitting 439 home runs, compiling a lifetime batting average of .340, being named the American League's Most Valuable Player three times, and being elected to the Baseball Hall of Fame in 1939.

His baseball career was ended on July 4, 1939 and he expressed his words of gratitude at Lou Gehrig Appreciation Day to thousands of fans and fellow players who had gathered to witness the end of an epoch. The fans knew he was sick and had been diagnosed with a horrible affliction, but few knew that the course of the next 2 years would be rapid deterioration of both upper and lower motor neuron function. Rapidly he would no longer be able to hit a curve ball, he would no longer be able to catch a pop up, he would begin to trip and fall, he would lose the use of his hands and arms, and eventually he would find it difficult to swallow, communicate, and breathe. The strike against Lou Gehrig was amyotrophic lateral sclerosis, someday to be known as "Lou Gehrig's Disease," and the final call would be fewer than 2 years later when he would succumb to the disease on June 2, 1941.

Amyotrophic lateral sclerosis (ALS) is one of a family of progressive, degenerative, neurologic diseases that affect movement, swallowing, and speech. It is a little-known but relatively common disease of the nervous system with no known cause and no known cure. Detrioration can be rapid with life expectancy generally to be about 2 to 4 years. In a study in southwestern Ontario over a period of years, the average time from diagnosis to death was 2.5 years. ALS occurs worldwide, though it has an unusually high incidence in Guam and southwestern Ontario, Canada. Worldwide, it affects 1.0 to 1.5 people per 100,000 population. Currently, approximately 30,000 people in the United States are diagnosed with ALS.

Even though the disease has been recognized for over 100 years and public awareness has been increased lately by calling it Lou Gehrig Disease, ALS is not well known. The short life span of most ALS patients is perhaps the principal reason for this lack of public awareness. It is not unusual for an individual to die within a few months of diagnosis of the disease. Also, patients tend to deteriorate rapidly, and their families have all the burden they can handle to keep the person functioning with some retained quality of life. Neither patients nor their families can spare much time and effort for public exposure and awareness. Typically, individuals with ALS are infrequently seen, infrequently heard from, and little societal interest or emotion is generated beyond the family.

Perhaps the association with Lou Gehrig, the Iron Horse, remembered for his lasting contributions to a popular American sport and for his heartbreaking farewell speech at Yankee Stadium, will elevate the condition in the public consciousness. We can only hope as well that ALS will be an expanded target of basic and clinical research.

ALS has a prominent role in this issue of our journal. An investigation of deterioration of vocal function in ALS is provided by Leeper and associates from Ontario, Canada. Description of the course of the disease by careful, objective means, as in this study, is an important contribution to understanding the nature of detrioration and possible signals and clues to the future. We also feature in this issue an elucidation of the communication disorders in systemic lupus erythematosus. This contribution, by M. Cherilyn Young, is almost a tutorial on the nature of this little understood condition, and this detailed article will serve as a fundamental resource for anyone wishing to learn about or conduct research on communication in lupus.

Our colleagues from the University of Arizona also have a contribution in this issue. Bayles, Tomoeda, and associates continue their investigation of Alzheimer's dementia, this time with a study that investigates performance on measures of communicative function in dementia.

In our Dialogue section, we have a provocative piece on clinician perceptions of limitations on ideal care in medical speech-language pathology. Much discussion is apparent at conferences and meetings about the effects of restrictions and limitations of patient services to people with chronic conditions, and this article reveals some interesting perceptions about trends in health care delivery. We invite your comments. Send a letter to the editor in care of this journal and express your perceptions, and we will continue the dialogue.

Under Clinical Notes we have two interesting reports. A cross-disciplinary effort from the University of Nebraska-Lincoln reports on improvement after fitting combined palatal and midfacial prostheses in an individual with extensive orofacial structural alteration. Also, we have discussion of certain issues related to maintaining hydration in nursing home patients with swallowing problems by Batchelor and colleagues.

CHAPTER 48

SURF AND SPACE

For I dipped into the future, far as human eye could see,
Saw the vision of the world, and all the wonder that would be.

—Alfred Lord Tennyson, *Locksley Hall* (1842)

L ittle did Lord Tennyson know. How could he have envisioned the
telephone, let along the Internet and the implausible advances in telecommunication that the dawn of the 21st Century would spawn. In 1842 advances
in science and technology included the first use of ether to produce surgical
anesthesia by Crawford W. Long, an American physician. In the same year,
Joseph Henry discovered the oscillatory character of electrical discharge, and
Queen Victoria would make her first railroad journey. Who could foretell that
a further dip into the future would include virtual journeys through cyberspace? Well, here we are.

The age of virtual reality, cyberspace, Internet, e-mail, and three-dimensional
VRML environments that mimic physical reality are upon us, even though
estimates suggest that only about 5% of the general population is computer
literate. Other estimates suggest that from 13.5 to 30 million people around
the world have access to internet services, and current growth rates predict the
size of the Internet will double every year for several years to come (*Cyberspace
Today, 3*, 1995). We have seen the future and it works, as someone has allegedly
commented.

Perhaps our wonder at the engaging dynamism of telecommunication will
appear quaint in the future. Certainly, fads and technology change. There is nothing so ludicrous as yesterday's fashion. As we live them, current styles seem ever
so apt. Whoever thought the pointy collars, bell-bottoms, and platform shoes
of the Sonny and Cher 1970s would be anything but ultra-chic? It is easy for
some to be pessimistic and gloomy about techno-change and about the future
in general. The lists of problems we will have to deal within the near tomorrow
seem to reinforce gloom. Publications such as *The Futurist* run a litany of future
problems. These include social discord, international tensions, fragile economies,
the drug crisis, the last elephant, chemical warfare, nuclear kamikaze terrorists,
militant vegetarians, and the danger of everyone turning into videonoids ("We
have our TVs and our work terminals . . . let's stay home . . . forever.")

But we must put these morbid forecasts into historical perspective. By a
look backward we can see that immense fears of a hundred years ago included
dread that by 1920 there would be no trees because sufficient quantities of
alternative building materials were not available. Another 1890 forecast that
turned out to be a little off was that the emerging popularity of the automobile
would result in quiet streets. "All the crash of horses hooves and the number
of steel tires will be gone, and since vehicles will be fewer and shorter than the
present pair of draft animals, streets will be quieter and appear less crowded"
(Center, 1990).

Other blunders of forecasting have sobered us throughout history. Thomas
Tredgold, a British railroad designer, declared in 1835, "Any general system of con-
veying passengers—at a velocity exceeding 10 miles per hour, or thereabouts—is
extremely improbable" (LaPointe, 1985).

In another example 2 years later, the surveyor of the British Navy, Sir William
Symonds, declared the screw propeller useless for driving steamboats. "Even if
the propeller *had* the power to propel the vessel, it would be found altogether
useless in practice because the power being applied to the stern, it would be
absolutely impossible to make the vessel steer" (LaPointe, 1985).

But even acknowledging the perils of forecasting, a look to the future should not petrify us, but challenge and excite us. The erupting age of cyberspace and the Internet will no doubt be critical harbingers of modes of information exchange in the future. For professions that are nurtured by data exchange, as are so many in health care, this can be nothing but gainful.

So in this issue we plunge into the advocacy of getting wired. Judith M. Kuster has prepared a technical note for our readers on "Internet Resources for Medically Related Communication Disorders." The joy of this type of compilation is the joy of discovery. One link, one thread, leads to another, and we become enthralled with how much information permutes and is available to us. A necessary caveat of the Internet is that addresses, sites, and sources of information change without warning, and blind alleys are a requisite hazard of the cruise. Kuster and our reviewers have done everything they can to ensure the currency of this most unique resource list, but are not responsible for the inevitable changes that occur after submission.

Other contributions in this issue include a most needed study of dysarthria associated with unilateral central nervous system lesions from the Mayo Clinic, Rochester. Joseph R. Duffy and W. Neath Folger have provided this careful retrospective analysis of this disorder.

From Canada we have a study of the perils to language in 5- to 7-year-old children who were born prematurely. This study looks at language behavior in this at-risk population with some attentive and insightful interpretations.

A survey study by Barrineau and Frank reports frequency of assessment protocols for adults with traumatic brain injury. It is always interesting and informative to get a bit of a window into current clinical practice even though the window might be colored by culture and country.

Finally, a clinical note from Dworkin and Abkarian considers some quite specific and prudently recorded clinical procedures for treating phonatory problems in an individual who suffered closed head injury. Although, there may be several clinical paths to reach a destination, it is always useful to have a path thoughtfully blazed with specific treatment strategies spelled out. These authors do this, and provide a good deal of background information on the nature of the condition as well.

So welcome to a dip into the future. The Internet and cyberspace are an inevitable part of our horizon and the vision of our world . . . with all the wonder that would be.

REFERENCES

Center, J. (1990). Where America was a century ago: History as a guide to the future. *The Futurist,* Jan.–Feb.

Cyberspace Today. (1995, May 18).

LaPointe, L. L. (1985). Training in aphasiology: Windows in the crystal ball. In R. Brookshire (Ed.), *Clinical aphasiology* (Vol. 15, pp. 15–21). Minneapolis: BRK Publishers.

Tennyson, A. L. (1842). *Locksley hall.* New York: Frederick A. Stokes.

CHAPTER 49

ON BEING A PATIENT

What's it like to be ill? Our ability to imagine the illness experience and to empathize with those who are ill is severely limited. Until one is actually in the patient role, it is difficult to place oneself in the role of a patient.

—Morse and Johnson, *The Illness Experience* (1991)

I once had a wise and benevolently autocratic hospital director who taught good lessons about being a "patient." At weekly meetings of the department heads and middle administrators of all units, including custodial and engineering as well as those involved in direct patient contact, he would routinely read letters from former patients and their families that contained critiques and comments on how they were treated during the hospital stay. Some of the letters were critical. We were not spared the bad news. But most of the letters were positive and revealed specific examples and incidents of how families or loved ones were processed by hospital employees.

> The social worker lined everything up for us. We were worried about what to do after discharge, but everything was taken care of. And she asked a lot of questions about our home situation, in a way that didn't embarrass us at all. She was very professional.

> The physical therapist helped a lot. We're still doing the exercises and she laughed and joked with my husband about how to remember the right way to do it. It helped a lot.

> The doctor cured me. I was scared and feeling way down about what to expect. The pills have allowed me to get about my business. I felt the doctor really cared about me as a person and told me that I could go on picking pecans and catching shrimp for as long as I wanted.

> I asked a woman with a cleaning cart how to find x-ray, and she smiled, stopped her work and showed me the way.

> Speech helped. I couldn't sign my own checks or even ask for things at the hardware store after my stroke, but they helped me get that communication stuff back. You don't miss it until it goes. It was hard work but they always made it interesting. Those speech people gave me back some words but also rescued some of who I am.

These are typical excerpts from the patient letters. Our hospital director always made the same unfluctuating point, so repeatedly and clearly that it became indelible.

"For the most part these people are incapable of judging the quality of medical care they received in this hospital. They are not trained in medical or health care practice and are unaware of the criteria by which to evaluate relative effectiveness of health care delivery. But they *can* judge how they were treated as individuals. They *can* judge whether or not they were treated with courtesy, with dignity, and with compassion. And that, primarily, is how they perceive and judge the quality of the health care they received."

This is a lesson I think those of us in health care delivery must take to heart and nurture. One of the most pervasive consumer complaints about health care systems is the perception that "patients" are dehumanized, institutionalized, robotized, and stripped of identity and individualism when control is wrenched from them as they are cloaked in the cape of "patient."

This need not be the case. Many good exemplars exist where it is not the case. Yet it is easy to fall into the snare of routineness when assisting with the

137th modified barium swallow, the 43rd ultrasound evaluation for epigastric pain, the 200th peri-oral exam, or the 50th administration of the RCBA. But for the person being evaluated at that moment, this routine, this new role, may well be a first. Procedures need to be explained. Rationales need to be revealed and clarified. Questions need to be answered. Fears need to be calmed. Coalitions need to be established. The uniqueness of the individual needs to be maintained. Dignity must be preserved. And all of this needs to be interwoven with the most current, professional intervention that clinical art and science will allow. But the lessons of how "patients" are treated must never be allowed to erode. We must practice these lessions, teach them, and incorporate them into our value systems. We are reminded compellingly of this when we become "patients" ourselves and suddenly are thrust into a very different role in our health care environment. But it should not take this startling role reversal to remind us of this golden health care rule. Competent practice dictates that incorporation of these principles be intuitive and reflexive.

Gifted writers such as the neurologist Oliver Sacks (1984) have transcribed personal accounts of their experiences in attempts to jolt their peers into a new kind of awareness when interacting with "patients." The depersonalization of the process is captured remarkably by Sacks (1984) as he relates his own feelings of foreboding and alienation upon becoming a patient.

> *One's own clothes are replaced by an anonymous white nightgown, one's wrist is clasped by an identification bracelet. One becomes subject to institutional rules and regulations. One is no longer a free agent; one no longer has rights; one is no longer in the world-at-large. It is strictly analogous to becoming a prisoner, and humiliatingly reminiscent, of one's first day at school. One is no longer a person—one is now an inmate. One understands that this is protective, but it is quite dreadful too. And I was seized, overwhelmed, by this dread, this elemental sense and dread of degradation, throughout the dragged-out formalities of admission, until—suddenly, wonderfully—humanity broke in, in the first lovely moment I was addressed as myself, and not merely as an "admission" or "thing." (p. 46)*

Let each one of us be the health care professional who will be interpreted as the humanity that breaks in. The illness experience is far from routine. We are beginning to learn a little about it and counter some of these negative impressions divulged by health care consumers. Medical sociologists, psychologists, anthropologists, and health care professionals are busy examining aspects of the illness experience, particularly how it relates to improvements in models of delivery of health care. Enlightenment can come none too soon.

In this issue of the *Journal of Medical Speech-Language Pathology* we have empirical research, methodological investigation, and a rich array of case reports and clinical insights concerning people who were thrust into the role of "patient" at one time or another. We begin with an article on the differential repetition of emotional and nonemotional words by people with aphasia by Ramsberger. Next, a study of perceptual aspects of dysarthria associated with amyotrophic lateral sclerosis is presented by South-wood. Following that is an interesting comparison of the effectiveness of computer-assisted instruction with traditional teaching methods in neuroscience by Frank and Montgomery.

Finally, three diverse and clinically relevant case studies are presented. First, a description of the effects of lightning strike on speech motor control by Hartman and Abbs. Second, a description of some therapeutic insights gained from working with a person with dysphagia following cervical spine surgery is presented by Magoon and Nelle, followed by a report of bite block therapy in two individuals with oromandibular dystonia by Dworkin.

I trust that this issue of our journal will be of some help as you go about the fulfilling task of interacting with our fellow humans who have cognitive or communicative handicaps. I hope as well that we reflect for more than a moment on the illness experience, what it is like to be a "patient," and how we can make it less daunting.

REFERENCES

Morse, J. M., & Johnson, J. L. (1991). *The illness experience.* London: Sage Publications.

Sacks, O. (1984). *A leg to stand on.* New York: Harper and Row.

CHAPTER 50

FIRST AMONG GIFTS

Before the harp, before the flute, before the fiddle, before all the other instruments made by human hand, there was the voice.

—Earle Hitchner (1995)

You never know when you will run across brilliant rhapsodies to human voice and speech. Since our passions and livelihood revolve around the wonder of human voice and speech, no doubt we are keenly sensitive to their value. We become aware how easy it is for most people to take these gifts for granted and what anguish it can be to endure loss or impairment of them. They are easy to take for granted. For most, the struggle of acquisition is dim to memory, and the act of speaking has been automatized and as easy as pie for years. As a man with aphasia with whom I worked once expressed it, "I never realized . . . I never missed the water til the well went to hell. Can you help me to just comb out the woolly parts?"

So it comes sometimes with mild surprise to see others express concordance with our perceptions of the precious nature of voice and speech. Earle Hitchner is one. Here he is on the liner notes of a music compilation entitled *Celtic Voices: Women of Song*, not only extoling the virtues of the human voice but being absolutely eloquent and poetic in his praise for this gift. Says Hitchner,

> *It can become a bare murmur of prayer, the cooing lullaby of a mother tending her infant, the bellow of soldiers in battle, the impassioned whispers of lovers . . . , or the sweet shout of joyful triumph. The human voice can reach deep inside us as no other sound on earth, opening our hearts and minds to people and places distant or near, real or imagined, familiar or strange, and to thoughts that "lie too deep for tears. . . ."*

Thanks, Hitchner, for expressing it so well. For we know what happens when the gifts are displaced or disrupted. This issue of our journal contains some prime examples.

From the Mayo Clinic we have a report of the frequency, risk factors, and nature of aphasia following left temporal lobectomy. Lutsep, Duffy, and Cascino present data from a unique population that will help us convey more information about communication sequelae to patients who must undergo left temporal lobectomy and their families. Following this study are two unusual clinical notes. First, Dworkin and Arden present the case of a 24-year-old female with laryngeal lupus and profound dysphonia who failed to respond to conventional corticosteroid pharmacologic management. A previously unreported therapeutic approach for this problem, Isshiki I thyroplasty, produced improvements as measured by videostroboscopy as well as acoustic, aerodynamic, and perceptual analysis. From the University of New Mexico, Oelschlaeger presents a case study and review of herpes simplex encephalitis with associated cognitive and language impairment. In addition to the communicative and cognitive dysfunction presented, this report reviews pathogenesis, symptomatology, diagnosis, and medical management of the disorder. Finally, from France, Gentil and Pollack present a tutorial review of perceptual, acoustic, and physiological research that has been conducted on the dysarthria associated with Parkinson's disease. This review should be useful to both researchers and clinicians who have to deal with people with this particular neuropathology.

For many, December is a month that marks a season of gifts. We are reminded of the first among gifts by Hitchner. Voice and speech allow us to reflect the heart and mind. May we continue to learn about these precious heirlooms, particularly what to do when they are broken. May *your* gifts be abundant and gratifying this season.

REFERENCE

Hitchner, E. (1995). First among instruments. *Celtic voices: Women of Song.* Milwaukee, WI: Narada Media.

CHAPTER 51

GROWTH

In our springtime every day has its hidden growth.

—George Eliot (Marian Evans Cross), *Felix Holt, The Radical* (1885)

The act or process of development; the size or stage of development; the gradual change from simpler to more complex; augmentation; expansion; excrescence. All of these concepts and definitions attempt to capture a universal aspect of living organisms. Mollusks, algae, green sea turtles, and humans share phases of life devoted to gradual maturity. Some species, fruit flies or mosquitoes, for example, develop rapidly and have a relatively limited life span, greatly restricting their development of an identifiable popular culture or much in the way of performing arts. Others, such as the Huron pine, take a while longer to mature. In fact the oldest living organism on this planet is a 10,000-year-old Huron pine discovered recently in a purposely unrevealed location in the wilderness of Tasmania. What characterizes most growth and development is the gradual nature of the process. The "every day hidden growth" belies the process, and just as we fail to perceive the movement of the hands of the clock, we underperceive the dynamism of human growth. It takes careful longitudinal measurement or a rarely visited aunt to observe, "Your son's grown a foot since last summer," to strike our awareness of accumulated growth.

Humans have a fairly well understood pattern of maturity. The anatomists of the 16th and 17th centuries formulated normative patterns of growth and development even while tripping over some of the details. Marcello Malpighi refined the anatomical techniques used to study the structure of the tongue by boiling it and removing its horny layer only a few years after René Descartes illustrated and explained reflexive movement as arising from a flow of spirits from the pineal gland (Mazzolini, 1991).

What is not thoroughly understood about human anatomy is the interaction and degree to which growth patterns vary among the complex subsystems that subserve speech and oral-motor behaviors. Dynamic changes occur in the craniofacial-oral-laryngeal anatomy during the very time humans are absorbed with acquiring speech patterns and refining other complex oral functions. These developmental changes in structure are much more obvious when viewed cross-sectionally than when appreciated longitudinally, but understanding, particularly the idiosyncracies of developmental interaction across subsystems, is fundamental to an appreciation of what to do when these structures go awry.

With this issue we have a rare and elegant contribution, and in fact devote the entire issue to a review of development of the craniofacial-oral-laryngeal anatomy prepared by Ray D. Kent and Houri K. Vorperian from the Waisman Center on Mental Retardation and Human Development at the University of Wisconsin-Madison. In the words of one of the reviewers of this submission, "This is a magnificent piece of work. It is obvious that a major effort was undertaken to develop the document. I expect that it will be an important contribution to the literature, and I anticipate that it will be referenced frequently in the future."

We agree. The work of Kent and colleagues has blazed a trail from Red Lodge to the archival libraries of the world. As was recently stated in a letter of support for the nomination of Kent for Honors of the American Speech-Language-Hearing Association,

> *Ray Kent's career is characterized by excellence. His professional vita is replete with examples of this quality. His published work encompasses elegant variations on the theme of the relationship between speech and movement across a mosaic of disorders of human communication. His influence on the programmatic theme of the moment and speech is uncontested, and no scholar can ignore his work and expect to be taken seriously. The impact of this influence is international and is of such substance that there is no doubt in my mind that it will endure and be referred to by future scholars as classic.*

> *If there is a model that is the life-blood of this profession, yet is precious and scarce, it is that of the scientist-clinician. Ray Kent adheres to and exemplifies the highest standards of science and the scientific method and is a professional template by both example and advocacy of scientific ethics. While he has the reputation of being one of ASHA's leading scientists, he has never lost sight of the value of carefully fashioned research questions relevant to those tens of thousands of clinicians faced with the daily problems of making decisions that affect the quality of life of the communicatively impaired. Kent's carefully motivated research questions and his scholarly reviews, among his many other contributions, attest to the viability of the model of scientist-clinician. Ray Kent is a bridge between the laboratory and the clinic and fulfills that role as well as anyone in the profession.*

We couldn't agree more. We are proud to devote the entire Volume 3, Number 3 (September) 1995 issue of our journal to this most important tutorial contribution and hope that it helps reveal and elucidate the "every day hidden growth" of the craniofacial-oral-laryngeal domain.

REFERENCES

Eliot, G. (1885). *Felix Holt, the radical*. New York: Merrill and Baker.

Mazzolini, R. G. (1991). Schemes and models of the thinking machine. In P. Corsi (Ed.), *The enchanted loom: Chapters in the history of neuroscience* (pp. 68–143). New York: Oxford University Press.

CHAPTER 52

CLASSIFICATION

. . . the descended larynx explains why you can speak and your dog cannot.

—Bryson, *The Mother Tongue*, p. 12

Then why do we continue to exhort our dogs, "Speak! Speak!" laboring as they do with an undescended larynx? Human speech, animals, and classification systems may be related only tangentially but are drawn together in the wonderful world of research that aims to understand, explain, and create new knowledge. It is always a source of amazement to many of us when forces external to the clinical or academic environments attempt to direct our agenda by the critique that "too much time is spent on research . . . not enough on teaching." It apparently is unclear to some that, without research and the creation of new knowledge, we would have only old things to teach. Nearly always, the most active and committed researchers are the most highly evaluated teachers as well.

So we struggle trying to construct a research agenda, that may or may not be immediately applicable, and toil to interpret, conclude, classify, and make sense of our surroundings. This process includes judicious classification.

Classification has been one of the principle strategies for nurturing order and understanding across many disciplines. Arrangement, grouping, assortment, apportionment, labeling, and sorting are all synonymous processes that attempt to capture some order and organization from seeming chaos. We have struggled as well in human communication and its disorders and have achieved far from universal agreement on the terms or systems of classification that we must apply every day. The specialty area of neurogenic communication disorders is a prime example, and disagreements over labels and terminology have waxed and waned for years (e.g., *aphasia; apraxia/dyspraxia; phonetic disintegration; anemic aphemia; subcortical, conduction, motor, sensory, transcortical, slowly progressive, fluent, predominantly expressive, Broca's, Lichthiem's, nonfluent, transatlantic cable, Wernicke's aphasia*).

We, however, have not been the first to grapple with classification systems. In a recent book review that documented about four levels of reference to the following quote, the author (Currier, 1994) cited J. L. Borges in the *Manual de Zoologia Fantastica* who reported that a certain Chinese encyclopedia stated that **animals** can be divided into:

a. belonging to the Emperor
b. imbalanced
c. tamed
d. sucking-pigs
e. Sirens
f. fabulous
g. stray dogs
h. included in the present classification
i. who behave like lunatics
j. innumerable
k. drawn with a very fine camel-hair brush
l. et cetera
m. who just broke a vase
n. who resemble flies from far off

Attempts at classification and understanding have to start somewhere. Despite the inherent quandry in classification, in research, and the continuing drudgery of the endeavor to interpret and make better the world around us, we continue the business.

This issue of our journal is another worthy example of professionals seeking to make sense of the disorders of interest to our readership. It is a particularly diverse and international collection of articles beginning with a detailed study of hypernasality in Parkinson disease from the Motor Speech Research Unit at the University of Queensland. This is followed by a study of motor speech programming and execution in myotonic dystrophy from the Interdisciplinary Child Neurology Center in Nijmegen, The Netherlands. A study of reasoning and the effects of concept training aquisition in aphasia is next from the Phoenix area in the United States. We then present an interesting and what should prove to be very useful dialogue on the subject of neurogenic stuttering. Ringo and Dietrich offer a detailed analysis and critique of neurogenic stutering along with a most comprehensive compilation of the extant writing on the topic. Nancy Helm-Estabrooks and Richard F. Curlee have been asked to comment on the topic and their insightful thoughts are part of the dialogue. The last article is a clinical note by a group of Canadian researchers on the topic of perceptual characteristics of hemilaryngectomized and near-total laryngectomized male speakers.

We can be comforted by the realization that our efforts at classification have been visited by others, by the value inherent in a descended larynx, and by the fruits of persisting research from our most talented colleagues.

REFERENCES

Bryson, B. (1991). *Mother tongue: The English language.* London: Penguin Books.

Currier, R. D. Five books on ataxia. *Archives of Neurology, 51,* 745.

CHAPTER 53

FRUIT BATS AND APPLES

So many new names were needed . . .

—Jespersen (1788)

When the first nonindigenous explorers of Australia arrived at Botany Bay in 1788, they found a world teeming with flora, fauna, and geographical features such as they had never seen. "It is probably not too much to say that there never was an instance in history when so many new names were needed," wrote Otto Jespersen from the deck of a square-rigged sailboat as he marveled at the land. (Bryson, 1990, p. 103)

This introduction to Vol. 3, No. 1 of our journal is being formed while on sabbatical leave at the University of Queensland, Australia, amid the incredible beauty and unique culture of a land that is filled with productive and brilliant people as well as koalas, wallabies, kangaroos, blue-tongued lizards, fruit bats (flying foxes), and a rainbow of lorikeets, parrots, cockatoos or threes, and attractive but dim-witted pink and white galahs. Lessons and insights are generated not only by interactions with staff and students in the labs, classrooms, and hospitals, but also by immersion into the culture and natural history of a novel environment.

Those of us with more than a passing interest in language are immediately intrigued by the uniqueness apparent in the lexicon (with a colorful and well-developed tradition of colloquialism and slang) as well as in the phonology. While our ears and our Wernicke's areas are gradually accommodating the difference in vowel and diphthong use, it will take a while to learn the rich lexicon with all its variations. Some phrases are easy and delightfully optimistic, such as the omnipresent "No worries," "Everything's apples" (in good order, under control), and "Good on 'ya." (approval, congratulations, way to go). Other expressions, however, will take a bit of familiarity and analysis:

"Next time you bung on a turn you won't sound like a drongo — I wouldn't come the raw prawn — dead set!"

(roughly . . . Next time you host a party you won't sound like a fool . . . I kid you not . . . honestly.)

"This is extra grouse tucker."

(This is very good food.)

So our understanding and appreciation of this land continues as we become enriched by the experiences of our daily ferry ride to the university as well as encounters with the green sea turtles of Heron Island and the parrots of the Lamington rain forest.

This issue of our journal brings a diverse and interesting set of topics to our readership. Cowell and associates use the medium of magnetic response imaging to shed pictures and light on prenatal risks to language and learning development. Solomon and researchers from the National Center for Voice and Speech at the University of Iowa report on tongue strength and endurance in a select sample of individuals with Parkinson disease. A study of tongue function in dysarthria caused by upper motor neuron damage is reported by Thompson and colleagues from Australia, and investigations of acoustic variability in hypokinetic dysarthria comes to us from Canada.

These data-based papers are followed by a technical note describing an interactive video station for use in nonliteral language rehabilitation, and a clinical note on a strategy to evaluate the ability to swallow capsules in people with dysphagia. This clinical note is accompanied by an invited comment from Edwards of the Mayo Clinic, Scottsdale.

So the first issue of the third volume of our journal, once again, is a rich array of tucker for cognition. Good on 'ya.

REFERENCES

Bryson, B. (1990). *Mother tongue: the English language* (p. 103). Ringwood, Victoria: Penquin Books.

Wilks, G. A. (1978). *Dictionary of Australian colloquialisms*. Sydney, Australia: Sydney University Press.

CHAPTER 54

THE BRAN

*Thank you for coming to our class and teaching
us things about the bran. The bran is very good to have.*

—Love, Craig

The above, unedited quote is from a thank you note penned by a second-grade class member at Kyrene de los Cerritos Elementary School in the foothills of South Mountain in Arizona. The teacher of this class, a particularly enlightened and dedicated professional, distinguishes her curriculum not only by careful presentation and integration of the value and richness of cultural and ethnic diversity but also by incorporation of a unit on disability awareness. These are important early lessons and budding values for young children. This class was particularly intrigued by the children's book, *First One Foot, Then the Other*, a story about the adjustment of a child to his grandfather's stroke and rehabilitation. Since they expressed strong interest in learning more about the brain, the teacher invited me to visit them, show some models of the brain, and talk about prevention of childhood brain injuries. I gladly accepted, and the above quote is representative of the responsiveness of these young learners. While they are obviously developing their spelling and syntactic skills, they have no shortage of enthusiasm and insight. (One particularly clever question was, "How does the brain get damaged if a rattlesnake bites you way down on the toe?") So I talked to them about the brain, urged them to wear helmets when bicycle riding, and distributed a new little green friend, "Artie the Brain Frog," who reiterated the lessons of prevention and care.

Yes, the "bran" is very good to have. But sometimes the inevitability of brain compromise leads to unique and puzzling communication and cognitive sequelae. In this issue of our journal, we have several intriguing articles on that topic. We begin with a feature by Hammen and Yorkston on respiratory patterning and variability in dysarthric speakers. This is followed by another study from the Washington group that has a good deal of clinical implication for the treatment of dysarthria. The examination and understanding of verbal repairs in dysarthria may offer insight for some very direct suggestions from the clinician. Another disruption of the brain, Alzheimer's disease, is studied longitudinally relative to possible deterioration of writing skills as the disease progresses.

In a Clinical Note, a Canadian group of researchers offers some description of the influence of long-term tracheostomy on developing speech and language in two children. Finally, in a Clinical Research Note McCall, Shelton, and Weinrich offer some worthy suggestions to both the clinician and researcher (these labels are not necessarily dichotomous) on collecting and managing data from therapy sessions with the brain-injured.

The "bran" and its disorders will continue to be a prominent feature of our concern. I hope you enjoy and find useful the fiber in this issue. Perhaps someday Craig or one of his classmates will join us in our pursuit of knowledge about this frontier of clinical science.

CHAPTER 55

VOICES

Joy is the sweet voice, joy the luminous cloud

—Samuel Taylor Coleridge

Sometimes voices lose their sweetness. Sometimes the joy turns to anguish when sweet voice is lost. The delicate balance of neural control of the exquisite mechanism of voice can be tilted by a wide range of nervous system pathology, as many of us are well aware. Vascular lesion, nervous system trauma, degenerative disease, and other evils, have the potential to wreak their ruin on the envelope of normal phonatory production.

This issue is special and comes very close to being thematic. In this collection, researchers and clinicians from several laboratories and clinics, and from disparate locations, present the results of their findings on phonatory and laryngeal dysfuction. Although methodologies and interpretations vary across papers, the streams of similarity and congruence are remarkable.

The first article, from the pastoral green of Wisconsin, is an exploration of phonatory behavior in several clinical groups of subjects with neurologic disorders. Kent and his co-authors present information obtained from men and women with amyotrophic lateral sclerosis, Parkinson disease, and cerebrovascular accident and contrast it with the performances of healthy geriatric subjects.

From near the Great Barrier Reef, Murdoch and colleagues examine phonatory dysfunction in upper motor neuron cerebrovascular disease. The somewhat surprising finding that many subjects in this investigation exhibited instrumental signs of *hypo* function is thoughtfully interpreted to indicate laryngeal "stiffness" among other possible explanations.

Following this is a series of three seminal articles on phonatory and speech features of Parkinson disease. The group based near the foothills and flatirons in Colorado (with collegial contribution from less elevated environs) has produced impressive programmatic research on this theme, with a significant influence on the direction of intervention for this disorder. First, Lorraine Olson Ramig and colleagues present the development of a therapeutic approach that focuses on voice therapy documented by instrumental and perceptual measures of post-treatment improvement and maintenance. This is followed by a report on the application of this unique intervention strategy with three cases of Parkinsonian Plus Syndrome, who exhibited severe speech and voice deficits. The third paper in this group is a careful acoustic and electroglottographic voice analysis during drug-related fluctuations in Parkinson disease.

The final paper in this issue addresses another critical area of the speech production system that affects voice: the structures and function of the velopharyngeal port. In a Clinical Note, Liss and her co-authors present a case for direct training of velopharyngeal musculature and a call for research on training procedures. In this paper a very useful physiologic rationale and review of sensorimotor control of velopharyngeal closure is included. This contribution is quite tutorial as the advocacy for direct velar training is developed and will no doubt prove useful for both sophisticated professionals and novitiates.

I hope this notably thematic issue provides fruitful information and luminous clouds of knowledge for our readership. The goal and joy of sweet voice is enhanced by these contributions, and we appreciate the sustained efforts of our contributors.

CHAPTER 56

THE GRASS

I am the grass.
Let me work.

—Carl Sandburg

This June in many of these places, the grass does its work. Not in the symbolic sense of Sandburg's intent, where the grass covered the graves and the memories of battlefields, but in the more literal and mundane sense of more yardwork. Summer chores are on us here as we try to balance our lives and keep track of housely and workly duties. Cleaning the sparkplug and giving a few cranks on the Briggs and Stratton can be a pleasant diversion or a dreaded chore. At work we continue the task of piecing together clinical and research information into a cohesive monograph designed to help those who practice or are interested in medical speech-language pathology. Increasingly it is becoming apparent that these work environments demand cooperation and teamwork across the professions. In this issue, for example, we have collaborative contributions from individuals in the meadows of medicine and dentistry as well as the field of communication disorders.

For starters, we present an article on differences in topic reference in the discourse of elderly men and women. Stuart et al. remind us that significant gender differences exist in narrative conversational topics. Females talk about people (themselves, other women, men), interpersonal matters (lifestyles, life's troubles), and household needs (food, clothes, decorations) among other things. Males talk about work (crops, animals, machinery) and sports or amusements (baseball, cars, cockfighting). These gender differences help define the normative range of discourse topics in the elderly so we can better judge the relevance of conversation in those with neurogenic disorders, for example.

The ability of people with aphasia to deal with synthetic speech is the topic of the second offering in this issue, from a group that has had much experience with the nuances, successes, and limitations of augmentative or alternative communication devices.

Language outcomes in children treated for acute lymphoblastic leukemia is covered in a third article, and 23 cases are described and explored in considerable detail. Following this article, Cannito, Murry, and Woodson look at the important area of psychosocial adjustment and attitudes toward communication in adductor spasmodic dysphonia before and after Botox® injection treatment. Finally, a technical note explores the use of inductance plethysmography to assess respiratory function and a clinical note describes a device for the management of velopharyngeal incompetence.

This is quite a varied offering, once again. I hope this issue captivates your attention and helps you in the clinical decisions that you must make. But when you finish, better get out there and get at that lawn. The grass is working.

CHAPTER 57

MARCHING

Ev'ry where I hear the sound of marching,
charging feet, oh, boy.

—Jagger and Richards (1968)

Marching. March. So here it is March, the third month of the year, the first number of Volume 2 of our fledgling *Journal of Medical Speech-Language Pathology*. We are marching into our second March and observing somewhat of a first anniversary of this venture. The acceptance of the journal as measured through the steady rise in subscribers has been encouraging. For most journals, the subscription list is comprised primarily of institutions, for the most part libraries. *JMSLP*, probably because if its reasonable individual subscription price, has attracted a considerable list of individual subscribers of practicing professionals in a wide variety of medical settings. In this day of library cutbacks and frugality (some international journals cost thousands of dollars per year for a subscription because of mailing expenses and dollar exchange rates), we are being asked repeatedly to purge university holdings of expensive, esoteric speciality journals. The *Estonian Archives of Toenail Discoloration* and other such works are increasingly vulnerable. It is refreshing to see our journal endorsed and able to be afforded by increasing numbers of libraries and institutions at a time of heedful scrutiny of library journal holdings. More invigorating is the growing list of individual and small department subscribers.

So we march into our second year, buoyed by a growing readership and an increasing number of manuscripts submitted for review. In this issue we again present an array of interesting and important contributions. Lefkowitz and Netsell follow their MRI atlas of speech production contribution of a year ago with another MRI study that correlates clinical deficits with anatomical lesions. Two intriguing case studies follow: first the speech-language findings in a child with the genetic disorder of trisomy 8 are presented; and next Paula Tallal and her co-authors report on a child with confirmed developmental bilateral damage to the head of the caudate nuclei. Next, a detailed analysis of acoustic parameters of phonation are plotted in a longitudinal study of Parkinson's Disease by Judith King, Lorraine Olson Ramig, and colleagues. Following that, the implications of naming deficit in multiple sclerosis are explored with a particularly cogent discussion of the neural substrates and the underlying bases of naming dysfunction. A detailed contribution to our Clinical Notes section follows in which McHenry and her co-authors demonstrate the clinical utility of the use of instrumentation to document changes in physiologic recovery across speech production subsystems in a person with traumatic brain injury. Respiratory inductive plethysmography, laryngeal and velopharyngeal aerodynamic assessment, and articulatory force measures were used to illustrate these changes. Finally, we present a unique purview on thought and language by Dr. Carl W. Olson, a philosopher who observes and comments on this complex topic from the perspective of his own aphasia. Dr. Malcolm R. McNeil provides some invited comments on this offering.

CHAPTER 58

TERM, HOLIDAYS, WORK

I remember summing up what I took to be our destiny ...
by the formula
'Term, holidays, term, holidays, til we leave school,
and then work, work, work till we die.'

—C. S. Lewis, *Surprised by Joy*

O ur friends and colleagues in Australia, in South America, and in other parts of the globe that lie south of the Equator, are now in the midst of summer, enjoying soda limonadas on the beach at Ipanema in Brazil or perhaps windsurfing off the Gold Coast in Queensland. Many of us in the Northern Hemisphere are reversed and are now dealing with either snow tires or snow birds, depending on our latitude or altitude. One thing is clear, this is a time of the year when holidays can alter our attitude, whether we are located down under or up over. While C. S. Lewis may have expressed our destiny in an oversimplified fashion, sometimes the formula of term, holidays, term, holidays, work, work, work can become a grind. However, when the work we have chosen is creative, rewarding, and provides a benefit to humankind, the process can be excruciatingly pleasant, despite toil and repetition.

This issue of our journal provides an adequate example of compelling and beneficial labor. We begin this issue with a much-needed tutorial on pediatric swallowing and feeding disorders. Most of us trained in the pre-swallowing era have felt the necessity to try to learn as much as we can about dysphagia and its clinical management. Much of this learning must be through continuing education, books, and review articles. Very little information is available on these special problems in children, and we are proud to present this foundation tutorial by Arvedson and Rogers who provide a synthesis of what is known about pediatric swallowing and feeding problems. A second article on swallowing, by Perlman and VanDaele, provides important normative information using technological advances in videoendoscopy and ultrasound.

Following swallowing are two rather extensive case reports. One documents language recovery in a case of severe head injury, and the other presents extensive objective documentation of the effects of voice treatment after bilateral thalamotomy. Two articles on phonatory features of unusual pathologies follow. Zraick and his co-authors, who have been engaged in an ongoing study of focal dystonia and its effects on speech and voice in a large sample of individuals with movement disorders, present a study of perturbation measures in subjects with spasmodic torticollis. LaBlance and colleagues present an unusual series of three cases of paradoxical vocal cord movement who were treated with botulinum toxin. Finally, a clinical note is presented in which Abkarian and Dworkin argue, "All we are asking, is give speech a chance."

Term, holidays, term, holidays, work, work, work. As is apparent from this issue, the work is quite obviously meaningful and fulfilling. May your holidays be restorative and gratifying as well.

CHAPTER 59

Brain and Red Rocks

This issue is being edited, fine-tuned, and assembled in the coral afterglow of the completion of the 23rd Annual Clinical Aphasiology Conference, held this year amid the majestic and mystical red rocks of Sedona, Arizona. One is reminded of the sustaining rewards of being a member of one of the professions devoted to advancing the clinical science and art of helping people who have disturbances of communication caused by brain faults and tremors. Perhaps geology and aphasiology are not so far apart. From Canada, Australia, The Netherlands, Germany, and all compass points of the United States (including the usual heavy representation from the cow-corn triangle of the Midwest) came professionals to the beauty of the Red Rocks country of Arizona. This year, as in all previous years, we presented new research, picked apart old studies, debated and argued during the ample discussion sessions, networked and exchanged ideas and complaints, hiked, fell down waterfalls, swam, relaxed, socialized, sampled fiery blue corn enchiladas and killer margaritas, laughed, and worried about the best ways to understand both the condition of aphasia and people with the condition. Once again from a forum of scholarly sharing most of us came away with a sense of satisfaction (*we can get some ... satisfaction ...*), challenge, ideas for new research or clinical strategies, and recharged batteries. Professional interaction at its very best—amid the dinosaurs and pictographs of the past.

Our journal, as well, can help fulfill this need for professional communication and interaction. We are surely one of Lewis Thomas' intricate social subsystems. With this issue, we once again present a variety of offerings designed to enlighten and inspire the members of this social and professional system who have chosen to try to do something about human communication and its disorders. We publish in this issue articles on swallowing problems associated with liver transplant, perceptual impressions of dysarthria, the effects of chronic otitis media on some aspects of language and hearing in children, a physiologic study of the interaction of jaw position and tongue actions, and a technical note on a sophisticated analysis system of speech distinctive features in alaryngeal speakers.

Just as our colleagues left the Red Rocks of Sedona with new insights and a sense of fulfillment and worth, our hope is that this issue of our journal will provide similar infusion.

CHAPTER 60

CROSSING TO SAFETY

The Spring of 1993 will serve as a temporal signal or marker of significance for many. Reasons for memory are assorted and individual, and events are always colored with the peculiar sensations and emotions associated with the circumstance. At the *Journal of Medical Speech-Language Pathology,* we have been heartened by the enthusiastic response of the professional community to the publication of our first issue. Not only has there been an expression of positivism for the quality of the content and production values of Volume 1, Number 1, but both the Editor and Publisher have enjoyed the fruits of initial acceptance by a rather significant increase in submitted manuscripts and subscriptions. Apparently in these times people just need to be certain that they are investing their minutes and money in a viable product. The response has been gratifying, and serves to underscore and reinforce the rationale and philosophy that guided the launching of this new venture. The uncertainty surrounding this beginning has given way, at least in small part, to a heightened sense of *Crossing to Safety,* with apologies to the late and revered American writer, Wallace Stegner.

Although our trek is just beginning, your comments and letters have been received as a measure of endorsement of both the need for and quality of our new journal. Many commented not only on the content but on the appearance and layout of the journal. A neurologist wrote, "The quality of the MRI reproductions is stunning. . . ."

From Japan, Dr. Minoru Hirano wrote, "Your new journal is unique and interesting. I believe it will be a good bridge between Medicine and Speech Pathology."

Several others noted the breadth of articles of interest to those in the medical environment, as well as on the production values apparent in the issue. To that point, I must express public gratitude to all of the people involved at Singular Publishing Group, Inc. A commitment to excellence permeates the philosophy and the implementation of this project, and special mention must be paid to the values and professionalism of Angie Singh, who coordinated the project, as well as to Marie Linvill, Ted Logan, Sandy Doyle, and of course to Sadanand Singh, whose imagination and vision actuated the notion. Thanks are also in order to the members of our Editorial Consultant Board for their efforts in soliciting and generating manuscripts for consideration. All new journals face a challenge in attempting to build a backlog of quality manuscripts to complete issues during the formative stages. We welcome your continued efforts to solicit and submit relevant work to us. With the gratifying increase in submissions after appearance of the first issue, this task may be less formidable than anticipated.

This issue, Volume 1, Number 2, continues the diversity and aptness of the first. We begin with a clinical case study of restoration and management of glottic insufficiency following laryngeal trauma induced by an equestrian accident. An article from an interdisciplinary group of Canadian researchers describes voice characteristics after hemilaryngectomy and near-total laryngectomy. Following that is a pair of studies on the theme of linguistic and speech breathing intactness and impairment in children who have undergone treatment for posterior fossa tumors. These studies come from the programmatic research on this topic from our colleagues in Australia. Following these articles are two on the topic of residuals of brain injury. From Nebraska, one on semantic organization, and from Iowa, a study is presented that reflects our increasing sophistication and understanding of disrupted cognitive processes after nervous system damage.

These are the offerings of Volume 1, Number 2. May they provoke thought, understanding, and perhaps enlighten the path of clinical management.

CHAPTER 61

OBJECTIVES, SCOPE, PHILOSOPHY

CONDUIT, ARCHIVE, WELLSPRING

An effective journal embraces several roles. As we define the objectives of this new journal we envision an evolution of its contributions and responsibilities. We hope to become a *conduit* that facilitates the creation of knowledge and the birth of ideas. A dynamic clinical science thrives on the accumulation and the sculpting of curiosities and creative thought. A journal can foster and convey these processes by the publication of original, useful research and contribute to the accumulation of data and ideas. We see ourselves as an *archive* for a growing clinical science. Tomorrow's scholars and clinicians should be able to consult records and trace routes and visualize patterns in the hypotheses, theories, and trends that are chronicled and preserved on our pages. Subsequent generations should sense the labor, and the blind alleys as well as the triumphs, of their predecessors. We are motivated also to be a *wellspring* of help for clinicians and practitioners. Not only are we interested in the genesis and accumulation of knowledge derived from a theoretical perspective, knowledge for the sake of better understanding and explanation, but we hope to be a refreshing source of clinical suggestion and direction for the many professionals engaged in the daily labor of making decisions of clinical management that alter the quality of living for the millions of children and adults with disorders of communication.

CONCEPTION

The *Journal of Medical Speech-Language Pathology* was conceived to fill what we feel has been a longstanding void and increasing need. We propose to focus on the issues, concerns, and needs of those professionals who are interested in human communication and its disorders as it is traditionally studied and practiced within a health care or medical model. Many specialty journals exist that address selected disorder areas within our disciplines, but there appears to be a genuine need for a publication that holds **the study and practice of medical speech-language pathology** as the unifying theme. Our journal will not be disorder specific but will span age, disciplines, and subspecialties in order to address the full spectrum of conditions and issues that contemporary professionals must face. Although the majority who practice in this realm will be speech-language pathologists, the proliferation of team approaches to rehabilitation, the blurring and melding of professional territorial boundaries, and the increase of cross-disciplinary collaboration in working with people with disordered communication make it probable that professionals trained in disciplines other than speech-language pathology will share and contribute to our objectives as well as enjoy the harvest of our travail. Many such professionals practice in hospitals, medical centers, rehabilitation clinics, private practices, or home health care delivery systems, but the transformation of world health care delivery continues to indicate that others outside these traditional venues of delivery will benefit from the information we impart. So while the primary targets of our journal will be speech-language pathologists, the related disciplines of neuropsychology, occupational and physical therapy, social work, nursing, counseling, as well as practitioners in the medical specialties of neurology, otolaryngology, plastic and reconstructive surgery, pediatrics, gerontology, and family practice will find information relevant to dealing with the communication disorders and related problems that plague the people seen in their daily practices. Our journal will be relevant as well to the school-based practitioner who must struggle to deal with the increase in medical or somatic components in the afflictions of the children and adolescents they encounter.

SCOPE
Age

We will not restrict our focus to any segment of the life span. Although the majority of the caseload in many medically based practices in communication disorders is drawn from the adult population, we see increasing need and attention to pediatric as well as geriatric issues. Mandated changes in the delivery of health care before and beyond the school-age population foretell increasing attention to infants with congenital malformation, chromosomal and genetic disorders, very low birth weights, and other severe medical problems. The specific effects of early medical problems on developmental and functional behaviors are an increasing target of clinical research. Numerous researchers and educators have spotlighted communication skills as one of the most critical needs of young children with severe disabilities. Further, the well-recognized greying and balding of world populations is documented by demographic studies that feature the elderly as one of the fastest growing cohorts, and disturbances of communication related to medical problems are among their most pressing complaints.

Disorders

While we anticipate that many of the manuscripts appropriate for our journal will concern **aphasia** and **related neurogenic disturbances** of communication such as **right hemisphere syndrome**, the **dementias**, neuromotor speech disorders (apraxia of speech and the dysarthrias), and the constellation of deficits that follow **traumatic brain injury**, we anticipate as well attention to disorders of **voice and laryngeal function, craniofacial impairment**, and any other disturbances of speech, language, or cognition that are seen in medically related practices. An increasing portion of the caseload of hospital-based speech-language pathologists is comprised of individuals with **dysphagia**, either neurogenic or related to other causes. Swallowing disorders are an important part of our evolving scope of practice, and we expect to provide an outlet for research and thought in this area. Special populations, such as **ventilator-dependent patients**, individuals with **spinal cord injury**, and those who have undergone **head and neck surgical procedures** or **tracheo-esophageal puncture** also fall within our realm of interest. Since our focus crosses the age span, **multiply handicapping conditions and developmental disabilities** that defy categorization but affect communication also will be appropriate.

Geography

To serve the needs of our readership and the profession, we intend our journal to be international as well as interdisciplinary. Important advances in the practice of medical speech-language pathology are evident in hemispheres other than Western. Although we will publish in English and no doubt draw many of our manuscripts from North America, we will attempt to avoid being ethnocentric, because we recognize that disturbances of communication recognize no national or cultural boundaries, and welcome work from members of the global community.

PHILOSOPHY

A philosophy and value that will anchor our foundation and permeate our publication will be adherence to high standards of scientific rigor. Although scientific motivations are not solely born of curiosity, we will do our utmost to ensure quality and eschew bias and subjectivity. Our editorial board and editorial consultants are selected because they are recognized as being among the most active and esteemed professionals in the world. Our peer review process will be anonymous, and editorial consultants will be blinded from the names and institutions of contributors. To maintain order and provide for a continuing reliable record, we will advocate adherence to the following principles as we evaluate material for publication:

Submissions should report specific, identifiable advancement in knowledge.

Arguments and interpretations should be logically consistent.

Research methods should be specific, testable, and detailed enough to be replicable.

Due reference to previous work should be cited.

Data-based submissions should conform to accepted methods of either group or single-subject empirical research designs.

Editor's Role

The role of the Editor-in-Chief in this process is clearly defined. First, the Editor will work with the Publisher to ensure that a high quality product is produced and distributed adequately. Next, the Editor's role will be that of a gatekeeper or guardian of our established standards to ensure that the criteria, constraints, and principles related to quality of content are upheld. Because we are an organ of communication and in such a role must interact with people on a daily basis to mold a worthy end product, we must be sensitive as well to human and interpersonal values. The Editor will advocate these values and no doubt will be called upon to assume the roles of arbitrator, counselor, promoter, messenger of doom, parent, and friend. Qualities and values that the Editor will attempt to bring to this journal will include tact, diplomacy, good judgment, appropriate humor, and professionalism. A scientific and scholarly journal is no place for wrath, dueling, politics, subjectivity, rudeness, sarcasm, abrasiveness, petty turf fights, or abusive language. Although these traits persist and appear as an invasive element in some academic and scientific circles, an important component of journal quality is the perceived degree of dignity and professionalism with which it goes about its business. We will value these qualities and will attempt to nurture them.

EPILOGUE

*Travel is fatal to prejudice, bigotry, and narrow-mindedness, and
many of our people need it sorely on these accounts. Broad,
wholesome, charitable views of men and things cannot be
acquired by vegetating in one little corner of the earth all one's
lifetime.*

—Mark Twain

*No one realizes how beautiful it is to travel until he comes home
and rests his head on his old, familiar pillow.*

—Lin Yutang

I write this from the 17th floor of the Montien Hotel in Thailand. The rising
sun is beginning to tint the exotic and beautiful Wat or temple that domi-
nates the view as I look down and across the city. This dazzling complex is
starting to hum with, from this height, bee-like monks in saffron and apparently even garnet colored robes scuffling their sandals around the complex.
They have been up, as most have at Thailand's 29,000 temples, since 4:00 am.
At 6:00 am they will have already logged an hour of meditation and an hour
of chanting as they wend their way through the neighborhood where the local
people will make merit by offering them food. At 8:00 am they will return to
the temple, sit together and eat breakfast, and then make a blessing for world
peace. So far, this daily blessing has only been partially successful.

On my desk is a complementary wooden bowl with a striking array of
four fresh Thai fruits. One of them is red, ovular, and hairy in appearance and
reminds me for some reason of my grandfather. It is a *rambutan* and when
its hirsute skin is squeezed or cut open with a knife the treasure inside is a
pale-colored, succulent fruit with a large seed. Complimenting the array is an
assortment of grape-like *sopodillas* (*lumat*) with a sugary but somewhat pun-
gent taste. Small, green-skinned tangerines I recognize, but have never tasted

such concentrated syrupy citrus flavor. Finally some tiny *kluey* (mini-bananas) complete the still life. Toto, this isn't Channing anymore.

This collection of essays has been a trip as well. As I have re-read them and traced travels, thoughts, and dreams over the past two decades, it has become apparent to me that they represent a personal trip not only to exotic lands on this great blue marble of ours, but also a genuine fruition of values. The recurring themes are perceptible and sometimes redundant, but what are ideas if one cannot repeat them and share them with others?

I am grateful for the opportunity that this collection has offered for self-expression. With any luck perhaps these essays have informed and even produced a grin or two. I am thankful and deeply appreciative as well for my colleagues, for my warm circle of friends across the globe, and for my beloved family. Soon it will be time to return home and rest my head on my old, familiar pillow. What a trip this has been.

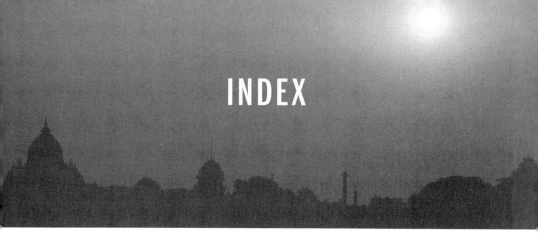

INDEX

absent presence, 46
Academy of Neurological
    Communication Disorders and
    Sciences (ANCDS), 146
advice, 121–124
ageism, 150–151
Age of Aquarius, 158
aging, 109–110, 126–127
American Speech-Language-Hearing
    Association (ASHA), 134–135
amyotrophic lateral sclerosis
    (ALS), 194–195
anguish, 118–119
aphasia, 107–111, 138–139, 142,
    162, 191, 226
apoplexy, 23
archive, 238
arthritis, 23
Australia, 40, 218

bad breath, 23
Banks, Joseph, 40, 41
Bauby, Jean-Dominique, 10–11
biographies, 173–175
brain, 221–222
brain damage, 170–172
Broca, Pierre Paul, 34–36, 92, 174–175
Broca's Brain (Sagan), 34–35
Buber, Martin, 7
Buckley, Kathy, 118–119
burnout, 26–27

Carlin, George, 14
cell phones, 43–47

censorship, 50
change, 133–135
children, feral, 65–70
chronicity, 109
Churkendoose, 5–7
classification, 213–215
Clinical Aphasiology Conference
    (CAC), 84–85, 178–179, 232
communication, 62–63
communication disability, 154
compassion fatigue, 25–27
complexity, 14–15
complimentary and alternative
    medicine (CAM), 22
conduit, 238
constancy, 134
conversation topics, 226
Cook, James (Captain),
    39–42
coping, 109–110
cultures, 153–156
culture shock, 99–102
cures, 21–23
cursing, 49–52
cynicism, 108

Demkina, Natasha, 54–55
denominator blindness, 2–3
development, 209–211
dictionaries, 149–151
diversity, 5–7
The Diving Bell and the Butterfly
    (Bauby), 10–11
dreams, 75–78

dysarthria, 159, 222
dysphagia, 230

education, 185–187
emotions, 118–119
empathy, 110
essay, 150
ethics, 134–135
eye puffiness, 23

familial change, 134
fear, 1–4
female professions, 18
female role models, 17–19
feral children, 65–70
First Asia-Pacific Conference
    on Speech, Language, and
    Hearing, 154–155
forecasting, 197–199
foreign language, 30–32
future forecasts, 197–199

Gall, Franz Josef, 36
Gardner, Daniel, 2–3
Gehrig, Lou, 194
gender, 18–19, 226
Goodglass, Harold, 187
growth, 209–211

hair balls, 21–22
head injuries, 170–172
health care, 167
helmets, 170–172
Hitchner, Earle, 206
hoaxes, 54–55, 69
holidays, 125–127, 230
hope, 71–73
human voice, 205–207
humor, 118–119

Internet, 198–199
irrational fears, 3–4
Israel, 45

Johnson, Samuel, 150
*Journal of Medical Speech-Language
    Pathology*, 228, 234–235, 238–241

language, 13–15, 29–32, 57–59, 150–151
language acquisition, 68
laughter, 117–119
life quality, 154, 189–192
locked-in syndrome, 9–11
loneliness, 61–63
Lou Gehrig's Disease, 194–195

Maori, 41–42
media, 2–3
mentors, 185–187
metaphor, 57–59
millennium, 146–147
mind-body connection, 72–73
mixed metaphors, 57–59
mobile phones, 43–47
motor speech, 129–131
Moxon, W., 92–94
Musée de l'Homme (Museum of
    Man), 34–36

National Aphasia Association
    (NAA), 138, 162
natural remedies, 22–23
neuromotor speech disorders,
    158–159
New Zealand, 40–42
night, 162
Nobel Peace Prize, 92

obscenities, 49–52
optimism, 71–73, 108, 110, 146

palindromes, 104–105
paranormal, 166–167
Parkinson disease, 224
patient interactions, 201–204
pediatric head injuries, 169–172
pediatric swallowing and feeding
    disorders, 230
peer review, 181–183
personal accounts, 161–163
pessimism, 108, 146
phonatory behavior, 224
preconceptions, 5–7
productivity, 88–89
profanity, 49–52

proverbs, 113–116
pseudoscience, 54–55, 165–167

quality of life, 154, 189–192

Ramón y Cajal, Santiago, 122–123
reductionism, 166–167
relational order theories, 14
remedies, 22–23
research, 214
reviews, 181–183
risks, 2–4
Roentgen, Wilhelm, 54
role models, 17–19

Sacks, Oliver, 203
Sagan, Carl, 34–36
schooling, 185–187
scientific debate, 123
sleep, 76–77
sleep apnea, 22–23
social isolation, 46, 61–63, 65–70
speech, 205–207, 223–224
speech-language pathology, 18
speech therapy, 10–11
splinters, 22
St. Anthony, 129–131
stroke, 162

Stroop test, 50
suffering, 118–119
superstition, 166–167
swear words, 49–52

taboo words, 49–52
Taiwan, 45
technology, 88, 198–199
telecommunications, 198–199
time, 87–90
tolerance, 5–7
translation, 95–97, 99–102

Vivaldi, Antonio, 142–143
vocabulary, 30–32, 150
voice, 205–207, 223–224
voice disorders, 191

wellspring, 238
Wertz, Robert Terry, 186–187
Wilson, Woodrow, 162
word play, 104–105
wound cleansing, 23

X-ray eyes, 53–55

youth, 125–127